The Hand from Behind the Curtain

The Hand from Behind the Curtain

Essays on Medicine, Fatherhood, Immigration —
and Other True Stories

FARHAN IMRAN, M.D.

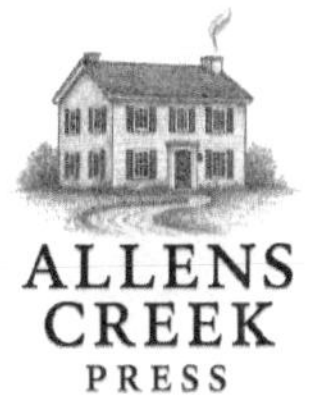

ALLENS
CREEK
PRESS

This is a work of nonfiction.

This book includes stories drawn from real patient experiences.
To protect privacy, names and identifying details have been changed.
In instances where individuals are identifiable, their consent has been obtained and is gratefully acknowledged.

ISBN: 979-8-9938824-0-6
Library of Congress Control Number: 2025923804

Publisher: Allens Creek Press, Rochester, N.Y.
Published in the United States of America

For

Zaina and Ziad

Contents

Essays by an Immigrant

Essays by a Divorced Single Dad

Essays by a Human

Foreword

By S. Amjad Hussain

"An exuberant bouquet of marvelous essays"

Cancer is a dreadful word. The mere mention of it brings forth the feeling of despair and helplessness. Despite great strides made in early diagnosis and treatment of many cancers, the dread still hangs over like a dark, ominous cloud on the afflicted. Hence, a book of essays by a cancer specialist would, one imagines, be a depressing read. I was pleasantly surprised that while most of the essays are about cancer and patients diagnosed with cancer, it is not a depressing book. In fact, it is a very enlightening and uplifting book.

Most physicians in the medical profession, thanks to corporate medicine that dictates so-called efficiency, have been forced to set aside the sacred principles of serving patients. Instead, they end up serving the corporate demigods. The cold and impersonal health care statistics are in fact patients with their tears wiped away.

Dr. Farhan Imran has the knack of making an ordinary encounter with a cancer patient significant and meaningful. Such an approach does not pull the rug out from under their feet but leaves them with hope. To be honest about a fatal disease and still leave the door of hope a bit ajar is a commendable trait. It is not the same as giving false hope.

While reading the book, I realized that it takes empathy and understanding to penetrate the stoic façade that many cancer patients develop. Behind the façade is always a vulnerable human being who is trembling with fear and uncertainty. It is the genius of the author to penetrate the façade and talk to patients in an understanding and sympathetic way. After all, patients not only need medicines to cure the disease or slow down its march, but they also need human touch and spiritual support in times of crisis. It takes time to take care of a cancer patient in a holistic way. The author strives to do that despite the time constraints placed on physicians by corporate medicine.

The practice of medicine is not only science but also an art. Blessed are the patients who are taken care of by doctors who are adept at practicing both. Here is an example of how NOT to deal with patients.

A Toledo native by the name of Ruth Hillebrand was living in New York City when she developed weight loss and a protracted cough. Upon investigation, she was found to have a large growth in one of her lungs. It was biopsied, and the result was a cancer that was beyond treatment. Her physician called her, gave her the bad news, said there was nothing more he could do for her, and hung up.

Though it was a terminal disease at the time, the cold and impersonal phone call shook her, and she remembered it to her dying day. In her will, she left 1.9 million dollars to the University of Toledo College of Medicine and Life Sciences with express instructions to use the money to train physicians and physicians-in-training in bedside manners. The Ruth M. Hillebrand Clinical Skills Center on the campus of the medical college bears testimony to how patients value good bedside manners. In this book, you will come across many stories where patients were served well by the author.

Throughout the book, the essays about cancer patients underline the fact that they are people in crisis. They must be treated with compassion and understanding. Even the most hopeless cases need a comforting human touch. I am impressed by how Dr. Imran expresses these traits in his encounters with patients. These essays are reflections of good bedside manners but also recognition of the sacred human bond between the patients and those who take care of them.

This book, however, is not all about cancer and its ramifications. It has essays about human relationships, philosophical musings, a lengthy but revealing dialogue between two women friends, one divorced and the other living in a miserable marriage. This essay expounds upon the status of the institution of marriage.

In the essay The Slow and Painful Death of Handwriting, he laments the deliberate neglect of teaching cursive writing in schools. I am also saddened at the young generation losing an age-old sacred connection with a writing instrument and an appropriate writing surface such as a stone tablet, papyrus, or a blank sheet of paper.

Dr. Imran was born and raised in Peshawar in the foothills of the Khyber Pass. Many essays in this volume reflect his upbringing in that part of the world. When he came to the US for medical training, he brought with him not only memories of a comfortable and privileged childhood but also the values his parents and society instilled in him. Many South Asian immigrants to the Western world live out their lives in a cocoon surrounded by the soothing and comforting mementos of their past. They live out their lives in relative isolation from the society in which they live. What good is a life, no matter how successful, when it does not touch and enrich the lives of our neighbors, co-workers, and even strangers?

There are another kind of immigrants that, upon getting off the plane, jump head on into the avant-garde culture of the host country, most culled from Hollywood movies. While they emerge cleansed of one's heavy cultural baggage, the skin tone and accent do not get exorcised through the cultural baptism.

Dr. Imran balances his own cultural heritage with the culture of his adopted country. This comes rather vividly through his writings. It is a tricky balancing act, but he comes through successfully.

In this book, Dr. Imran shows us how to live a full life, be attentive to his patients, have respect for the culture of other people, and live a happy and contented life.

Professor Dr. Sayed Amjad Hussain

Professor Amjad Hussain holds an *emeritus professorship in cardio-thoracic surgery* in the College of Medicine and Life Sciences and an *emeritus professorship in humanities* in the College of Arts and Letters at The University of Toledo. He is also an *award-winning writer* who has published numerous books on subjects as varied as history, culture, religion. For over 30 years he has been an *op-ed columnist* for the daily Toledo Blade and a number of other English and Urdu publications in the U.S. and in Pakistan. In 2011 he was given the *Touchstone Award of the Press Club of Toledo.* Recently in May 2025, during the university's undergraduate commencement ceremonies he received an honorary *Doctor of Humane Letters (honoris causa).*

Preface

My last patient for the day yesterday happened to be a long-distance runner. He was seventy years old and still running about twenty miles a week.

We instantly connected when we discovered that we were training for the same upcoming half marathon in three months. When you sign up for long-distance races, they put you into your age category.

As you age, the number of runners competing in your age category starts diminishing. The number of participants in the sixty-plus age category is only a handful of runners.

But at that age, just participating in and then finishing the race seems to be such a significant accomplishment that the time you take to finish the race doesn't matter as much. I told him he was an inspiration to me, and I wanted to run marathons in the highest age category someday, just like he was doing.

He had an accomplished career as an electrical engineer and retired as an executive at a reputed national company. He told me that long-distance running had taught him the strength and the discipline to face any challenge in his life. I couldn't agree more.

We talked about how one has to have some level of masochism to enjoy long-distance running and aim to keep running well into old age. Not only does it prepare you to face any adversity that life may throw at you, but several other abilities also stem from your acquired skills.

You do a lot of thinking while running straight for anywhere between one to five hours. Yes, you may listen to an audiobook, a podcast, or a long playlist of your favorite music.

Still, there comes a time when your body is moving, your ears are listening, your eyes are seeing, but you are thinking about something completely different.

Your mind wanders on and on. You get into this zone of detachment of the mind from the body. The brain becomes a playground for thoughts, ideas, emotions, and feelings.

During these moments, the idea was born into my mind that I ought to write these thoughts down.

After all, a thought only thought might disappear in thin air in just a few moments, but a thought written down on paper might survive for centuries and may have the power to change the world.

I started writing some of my thoughts. I wanted to share them with the world. Many people I talk to tell me they write, but only for themselves. But I am different in that way.

I wanted to write to display my thoughts to the world.

More than anything, I wanted to leave my thoughts for my children to read someday and tell those stories to their children, my grandchildren.

Maybe my words would lie somewhere in a drawer on a discarded study table. When it is being disposed of to a Salvation Army donation center, a great-great-grand-child might save the pages and stick them into their study folder to read them and get to know me and my thoughts after I am long gone.

I put together a website and started posting some of my essays online. To my surprise, they were received quite well, and in a short period of time, my essays were read by thousands of readers, which encouraged me to share more thoughts and tell more stories.

From a very young age, I saw myself as someone who had an opinion about anything in life. Even when I was in elementary school, I would ask a lot of questions and think about everything.

As I grew older in my teen years, I found myself giving advice to my friends even without being asked. I would be the kind of kid who sits in on adult conversations and, instead of staying quiet, voices his opinion and is sometimes asked to shut up, but other times, the opinion is better received.

When I was in my twenties, my father routinely started asking me to participate in discussions regarding family matters, finally giving me some validation.

Then, I became a father to a girl and then to a boy. These bundles of joy.

As they were growing up, I always thought to myself how lucky they were because I would impart unparalleled wisdom to them. Teach them every step of the way and tell them what to do when faced with any challenge in life.

In my mind, so many people had benefited from my opinions, including my friends, family members, patients, and colleagues. My children would be so lucky to have me guide them through any difficult situation that they encounter in life. They would have unlimited access to my insightful opinions and invaluable advice.

I did not see it coming, though, that when these little bundles of joy start growing up, they develop their own opinions, which may not always align with your suggestions. They simply may not be interested in what the opinionated father has to say to them.

As teenagers, it is not unusual now that when I give them advice on some important matter, they turn around, and even before I have finished saying what I'm trying to say, they will respond with "Did I ask?"

But it is challenging, sometimes impossible, to not like something that your children say or do.

This retort, "Did I ask," was so beautiful and endearing that I chose to give this name to my blog. This book you are holding is a compilation of the essays I have published on my blog for the last few years.

They say that every man's thoughts and behaviors are the average of the five people he spends most time with.

Similarly, a writer's writings reflect different aspects of his personality and what kind of life he is living. In my life, I wear several hats and play several roles portrayed in my writing.

The foremost would be my occupation. I am an Oncologist, and for the last ten years of my life, every single day, I meet with and make life-and-death decisions with patients who suffer from cancer. I become a vital part of their life and more pertinent than some family members.

Every patient's case is a story. Some stories are so moving and touching that not telling them would be shameful. Doctors are under stringent restrictions nowadays to guard the privacy and confidentiality of patients, and rightly so; hence, the names and other identifying information of the patients have been altered.

Every story in this book is a true story. However, in order to protect the privacy of patients, the names, ages and other identifying details have been changed. On some occasions, the characters are composites.

Creative license has been practiced where some details may have been altered or dramatized to make them more readable, but this compilation does not contain works of fiction.

Some of the stories involve serious and medically sensitive themes such as death, end-of-life illnesses and grief which might trigger unwanted emotions in some readers' minds. Therefore, reader discretion is highly advised.

Another aspect of my personality which influences my writing is that I am an immigrant.

Humans have migrated from one part of the world to another since the beginning of time. That is thought to have been the way of life for all humans for centuries when we were hunters and gatherers and changed only when humans learned agriculture. In today's modern world, migrations happen all the time.

I was born in northern Pakistan in the ancient city of Peshawar, part of one of the original human civilizations around the Indus River.

I immigrated to New York in my twenties to train and practice as a physician.

I went through and am still going through the different experiences, both good and bad, of being an immigrant, and you will see some of that reflected in some of the essays.

There was a time when I was a happily married man, but then 'life happened' and due to some unfortunate and irreconcilable differences, my wife and I had to go through a divorce.

This was a particularly difficult time for both of us and our two beautiful children.

The turn of events led me to assume the role of a single father I had least suspected. It has been a challenging role and, amongst other things, has given me immense respect for all the single parents in the world. Single moms are more common in any culture or society than single dads.

Still, the role is unquestionably challenging for everyone, a bit more difficult for the dad than for the mom, some might argue.

Consequently, my experience has colored some of the essays from the perspective of being divorced and as a single parent.

Behind all the identities we acquire in this world, at the end of the day, we all are humans. Beings that think, feel, perceive, and express. Some of the essays you will read cannot be categorized into any particular genre but are pure thoughts and feelings being conveyed from the mind of one human to another.

Please allow me to express my gratitude to you for choosing to read my stories. Now it is time to grab that favorite beverage of yours that pairs best with reading, and I hope you enjoy reading these essays as much as I enjoyed writing them.

Farhan Imran, MD

Essays by a Doctor about his Patients

The Hand from Behind the Curtain

I have been working at this hospital for almost two decades. This is where I grew up as a physician. After my home, I have spent most hours of my life within these walls and walking around these hallways.

The hospital is situated in the northernmost part of the country along the coastline of Lake Ontario. On a sunny, clear day, you can imagine the breathtaking view of Toronto's skyline from the top floor of the building.

The hospital used to have two main buildings, but a few years ago, the administration decided to erect a third building, which is a state-of-the-art facility.

When the construction of the building was near completion, we were given a tour of the facility. We were amazed by how large and well-equipped the patient rooms were.

The patient rooms were exorbitantly spacious and outfitted with comfortable furniture for family members. Each room had a beautiful view, surpassing any that local hotels offered.

Walking through the yet unfinished rooms, I made a comment that my colleagues thought was in bad taste. "Take a good look. Whoever amongst us ends up living in Rochester long enough, it is a good possibility that we will die in one of these rooms."

It was a Monday, the beginning of the workweek. I looked at the list of cancer patients that I had to round on. Although most patients were on the oncology floor, others were distributed throughout the hospital, including the Old Building and the now fully operational New Building.

I first started rounds with the residents and medical students in the New Building. I took some of the new residents to the break area to look at the views of the lake and downtown through the large windowpanes.

After seeing a few patients, we headed to the Old Building. Amongst others on my list was Mark, who was my patient suffering from stage IV lung cancer but doing exceptionally well on immunotherapy.

Unfortunately, he was now admitted with shortness of breath, and we were debating whether it was from pneumonia, medication-induced pneumonitis, or both.

Mark had an auto repair shop on Dewey Avenue, trades in luxury cars, and often joked that if I cured his cancer, he would get me the best car deal possible.

I used to tell him that I was perfectly happy with the car that I was driving, to which he always quipped, "Doc, is that your way of saying that you don't want to cure my cancer?"

We walked into Mark's room. It was tiny (compared to the rooms in the New Building), and his two sisters were by his bedside. I had three students with me, so seven people were in the room, including Mark and me. We were clearly having problems fitting in.

"How are you feeling, Mark?" I asked.

"My breathing is so much better but still not yet back to normal. I would have liked to stay another couple of days in the hospital, but I really want to get the hell out of here," Mark replied.

"But why don't you stay in the hospital until your full recovery, Mark? Why the impatience?"

"Well, have you looked at this room? This is smaller than the bathroom at my house. The last time I was admitted to the hospital, I was in a room in the New Building, and that was like a room from the Ritz Carlton. This one is as if I'm in a Motel 6!" he complained.

"I understand what you're saying, Mark, but the size of the room does not reflect the quality of care you are receiving. The nurses are doing an excellent job, and your treatment is working just fine," I pointed out.

"I understand that Doc. I know this is not the priority, but I would appreciate it if either I could go home as soon as I can or if you could pull some strings and move me to the New Building," he persisted.

"OK, well, I will see what I can do," I falsely promised.

Next up on the list was a patient I would see for the first time. The resident presented her history to me. She was newly diagnosed with metastatic bladder cancer, and while she was informed of the diagnosis, this was the first time she was going to meet an oncologist.

I had to tell her about the incurability of the disease and that she had no more than another few months to live. This would be one of, if not the most, important conversations of her life for which I wanted to create as comfortable an environment as possible.

However, as I walked into the room, I realized that it was one of the few rooms in the Old Building that was a shared room, meaning there was another patient in the same room.

In administrative meetings, I heard that they were trying to convert all the rooms into private rooms, but they did not yet have the capacity to do that. Many hospitals in the country now have private rooms, and shared rooms are now considered a thing of the past.

It was a room about half the size of the rooms in the New Building. There were two beds, which were separated from each other by a flimsy curtain. Sue, our patient, was in the bed closer to the entryway. The nurses were administering medications to the other patient, also a woman. There was hardly any room for additional people.

I pulled up a chair and set it up as close to Sue's bed as possible. The residents had to stand in the corners of the room.

I pulled the curtain a bit more to give Sue as much privacy as possible. I asked her if she had any close family members or friends with whom she wanted to be part of the conversation.

It turned out that she was close to only one of her daughters, who, because of her own medical issues, could not be there. Sue had to partake in this conversation all on her own. I started telling her about scan findings and pathology reports and explained her diagnosis in detail.

She appeared impatient and eventually asked the inevitable. "How long do I have to live, doc?"

I wished there was someone with her before I gave her the answer. "If we don't do any treatments, you may have another few months to live, but with treatments, if they are successful, I'm hoping we could be looking at a year or two as a best-case scenario."

Sue's hands started trembling, her mouth appeared dry, and everyone in the room could feel her palpitations. She broke down into tears that rolled down her eyes.

As I looked around the room to find a tissue box, trying desperately to do something to comfort her, I saw the curtain move. I saw a hand emerge from behind the curtain, trying to reach for something.

There was the IV stand carrying the infusion bags, and for a moment, I thought it might be one of the nurses trying to reach it to stop the infusion. The hand kept exploring and finally reached for Sue's hand and held it firmly.

Then, the other hand removed the curtain entirely, and I saw the other patient, not moving from her bed but having reached out to Sue to ease her pain and sorrow.

At that moment, no sympathetic words could replace the loving touch of a fellow human being.

Here I was, worried about the lack of privacy afforded to Sue at the time of having such a difficult conversation. Part of me worried about the HIPPA laws ingrained into our minds over the years.

I came to find out that Sue and Jenna had been in the same room for a few days now, had become good friends, and were sharing each other's worries through their illnesses.

Sue was discharged from the hospital soon afterward and now follows up with me in the clinic. Her cancer is responding to chemotherapy, and she has a decent quality of life. She tells me that she is still in touch with Jenna. They don't live too far away from each other and meet regularly.

Loneliness amongst the elderly and the ill is an epidemic that the US Surgeon General declared to be a central issue in his advisory statement in 2023. What leads to loneliness? There could be multiple possible explanations.

But to me, society's emphasis on individualism is one reason behind rising rates of loneliness. The individual is at the top of the agenda.

In the world of family law, as children and the elderly are being helped in the form of preventing abuse, they are separated from their families and put into foster and nursing homes, respectively.

In the world of rising women's rights, they are being burdened with two jobs of employment as well as rearing a household, often alone as single mothers, driving them to the brink at times.

The nuclear family living together happily is being destroyed by having the children leave the house upon adulthood in search of their own livelihood. Grandparents are being left alone in the guise of autonomy and independence.

Next-door neighbors are estranged in pursuit of privacy and seclusion. Work-from-home jobs are more convenient, but the bonds with work colleagues are becoming increasingly scarce.

A private hospital room should not be considered a luxury in today's world. Don't get me wrong. If I'm admitted to the hospital, I want a private room too.

However, the days when there used to be a ward with multiple patients in one large room together, although inconvenient, built a sense of community.

Now, you have more privacy and comfort, but it comes with another unwanted, uninvited, ominous visitor – loneliness.

Lucky The Duck

There is no news that one can hear about oneself that is more dreadful than being told that you have cancer. The mind shuts down for a few minutes. No matter what the doctor is saying, the words do not register.

It is like in the movies. Except, the only difference is that the scene passes in the movies, and there is a happy ending. Not in real life.

The scene has just begun, and the ending could very well be anything but happy. Such was the state of mind of Rick when he heard for the first time that the reason he could not get any relief from constipation, no matter what remedy he tried, was that there was a golf ball-sized tumor sitting in his colon.

Having just entered the eighth decade of his life, Rick had led an otherwise happy and fulfilling life as a high school biology teacher. He was a simple and kind man with the neat and scholarly appearance you would expect from a teacher.

His simplicity was evident from the ballpoint pen nicely tucked into the front pocket of his shirt that he pulled out along with the little notebook that he still used, in this electronic age, to jot down important dates and to recall doctor's appointments.

He had married the love of his life, who, over the years, had taken on the role of redirecting him, either with short two or three-word sentences or sometimes simply with her gaze, every time he had a lapse of cognition.

The surgeon felt like an angel descended on earth sent by God. She had used her skill, and it seemed nothing less than a miracle when she told him in the recovery room, as his deep slumber of anesthesia was wearing off, that she was successful at removing the giant tumor.

However, the cancer had spread to a number of surrounding lymph nodes.

There was a high chance of the cancer coming back in the next few months if he did not go through brutal chemotherapy in an attempt to kill any remaining cancer cells in the body. For that, he had to see a medical oncologist, and that was when I met him for the first time.

"You will go through three months of chemotherapy. It will be hard, but you should be able to get through it," I explained.

"Will that make sure that the cancer will not come back?" he asked.

"There are no promises, unfortunately, but we will get scans of your body every few months for the next five years to look for any signs of cancer coming back," I replied.

Disappointed at the lack of guarantee of a cure, he looked into my eyes, trying to find hope, only to find my attempt at making a poker face.

He finished chemotherapy without any major side effects, and we started obtaining scans every few months. Scan after scan showed no sign of cancer.

The three of us would sit down, and after discussing the scan results, we would talk about each other's lives and share stories of the past few months since the previous office visit.

This is when, for the first time, I heard about the story of 'Lucky the Duck.'

Rick got home a few days ago after his cancer operation and was recovering in the comfort of his home. He was walking around the house but not yet going out or lifting anything heavy.

One day, as he stood in his living room, he looked outside his glass windows and saw the backyard covered entirely with snow. The swimming pool was covered to protect it from the harsh winter.

His eyes suddenly caught on a small round object sitting on top of the swimming pool cover. His curiosity compelled him to walk outside carefully to see what it was. As he got closer, he found out that it was actually an egg.

As a biology teacher, he was used to handling eggs. It was a routine for him to incubate eggs as biology projects to teach his students about the life cycles of various birds.

With no way of knowing whether the egg was fertilized or not, he brought it inside anyway. It may even have been frozen, terminating any signs of life inside the shell.

Nonetheless, he took it to the basement, where he had the incubator that he used in the classroom, currently collecting dust since he retired. He placed the egg near the heating rod, adjusting it to the exact temperature required for the egg to hatch, 101 degrees Fahrenheit, as he had taught his students for several decades.

Every day, Rick would come to the basement to check on the egg, not knowing whether it would hatch. Each day he would turn the egg just as the mother would in the nest. When nothing happened for a couple of weeks, he could have just picked it up and thrown it in the trash bin - but something in his mind told him to keep watching.

On the twenty-sixth day, when he walked into the basement, he saw a small baby duck chirping lightly, sitting amid the cracked eggshells. It was so tiny that it could barely walk and open its eyes. Rick smiled at the memory which he described as "cuteness overload." He named the duckling "Lucky."

Not having grown up in a pet-loving home, I don't usually know much about different pet animals and the nuances of taking care of them. "Is a duck a usual animal to keep as a pet?" I asked with genuine intrigue.

"No, it's not. But nothing is stopping you from giving a duckling a loving home if you want to," he replied. "But I have to be honest. I don't really want any animal control authorities to find out, so please keep this story to yourself. I don't know what their rules and laws are. I don't want to lose Lucky."

Lucky ate what usual bird pets eat: Rice Krispies, cereal and worms. He liked to sleep off and on just about anywhere in the house but often in the bed made out of an old cardboard box. He came and sat in his parent's laps when he felt like it. He sat in Rick's shoes to greet him when he arrived home from the grocery store.

Lucky loved to stay indoors and be warm most of the year. He became a family member featured in all Christmas photos. His birthday, aptly named hatch-day, was celebrated each year.

Rick thought of Lucky as a therapy duck. As Rick healed from surgery and the effects of chemotherapy, Lucky sat with him, thus bonding and imprinting. Rick relaxed, as did Lucky when he held him.

The only thing Mrs. Rick did not seem thrilled about was that Lucky could not be potty-trained, so the entire house needed to be constantly vacuumed.

Still wanting to see the optimistic aspect of the situation, she told me that is how she got her daily exercise.

Somehow, it appeared that Rick's journey of going through cancer ran in parallel to Lucky's life. Lucky was born and adopted, essentially given a new life at around the same time when Rick's oncology team declared him to be cancer-free after his surgery.

Rick's cancer remained in remission for a couple of years when, during a clinic visit, I had to break bad news to him.

"Your scan is showing a nodule on your lung. It could either be cancerous or not, but we cannot find out because it is too small to stick a needle into it for a biopsy. We can only repeat the scans every three months and see if it grows or disappears. If it grows, we are in trouble; if it goes away, we are all set." I explained.

"But do you know how hard it is to live with this uncertainty, Doc?" he responded.

"I know, and I wish I could help with that, but I can't. Nobody can," I replied.

Those few months were very difficult for Rick. Those were the days when Lucky also went through a life-threatening incident.

Lucky ventured outdoors each day where he would fly away and always come back in an hour or so. One morning, Lucky did not return. Three hours passed, then four, then six. The anticipation increased. Rick thought of at least a hundred scenarios of how Lucky may have already died.

That is when his neighbor called to inform him that he had found Lucky in his yard. He rushed to bring the duck home and found him lying feebly under a tree.

Not only that, but several of his feathers were chewed out, and there was also a sizable wound on his side. He instantly realized that the neighbor's dog, Rover, a golden retriever, had bitten Lucky, and while escaping for his life, he got stuck in the bushes.

Rick brought Lucky home and nursed him for the next few weeks. Lucky did not quack or fly for three weeks. While his wound healed, not all of his feathers grew back. Consequently, Lucky never left the front yard whenever let out after this incident. It was as if he was scarred for life. But all's well that ends well, I guess.

He was still alive. Rick had a similar kind of relief when I told him at a visit that his lung nodule had disappeared on a follow-up scan.

At the end of five years of follow-up, I told Rick, "This far out, the chances of your cancer coming back are now down to the point that you don't need to see me anymore."

Happy and relieved to hear that, he invited me to his house to meet Lucky. Lucky was even more loving and beautiful than what I had so far construed him to be in my imagination.

As I was leaving the house, looking at Rick, cured of his cancer and Lucky having endured a number of potentially life-ending incidents, a thought struck me.

"Why did you name him Lucky?" I asked Rick.

He responded matter-of-factly. "Because it was his good luck that I found his egg before it was destroyed."

Was Rick lucky for Lucky, or was Lucky lucky for Rick? Maybe Rick was the one who was lucky to have survived the cancer, and in some spiritual realm, this was all because of his act of kindness towards Lucky.

Mr. Hendricks

If my grandfather were alive, he would be the same age as Mr. Hendricks. Seventy-eight years old.

That's why when I first met him, he introduced himself as John, but I preferred to call him Mr. Hendricks. That's how I was taught as one of the ways to give respect to the elderly.

The "American" way is to call someone by their first name if you have some level of closeness to them and that's what he prompted me to do a couple of times: "Call me John."

But I preferred to abide by the mannerisms taught to me by my upbringing and chose to give him respect by calling him Mr. Hendricks.

He was referred to me for anemia. "You have half the amount of blood in your body compared to what you should normally have. That's why you feel so tired and short of breath all the time," I explained. "The fancy word for your disease is Myelodysplastic Syndrome but in easy terms let's say that if your body was a car, your gas tank would have a hole in it and your fuel gauge is on Empty all the time."

He seemed understandably alarmed. "Well, how do we fix it then?" He inquired with cautious optimism.

"This is an incurable disease for someone your age. We can give you chemotherapy which may slow it down, buy you a few more months or years to live, but there is nothing we can do to completely get rid of it," I responded.

"How long do I have, Doc?" he asked the ultimate question.

"Most people in your situation will have another year or two to live. With treatment that is. If you choose to go without treatment, it could easily be less than six months," I answered.

"Do some people choose not to do any treatment at all?"

"Yes. A few people will say that if a disease cannot be cured and if they feel that they have lived a good life and are ready to go, they might choose not to go through chemotherapy." I explained.

He decided to get his treatments.

He came to the cancer center on a regular basis. Within a few visits, he became a favorite among all the staff.

Decades of life experiences had turned him into an extraordinarily polite and kind man. He had a remarkable ability to pierce through any interpersonal barriers and get acquainted with the personal issues of several nurses and staff members.

This was aided by the fact that he was a handsome man. Always sharply dressed and carrying his grey hair and wrinkles like a seasoned movie star.

I got to know him more as the months passed by. He went through a bitter divorce earlier in life but then fell in love with Kelly who was eighteen years younger.

They were married now and seemed to have a very happy and content life. Their affection for each other was visible in each word and gesture.

Such was their love for each other that upon hearing the news of him having an incurable illness, Kelly could not stop her tears and although he was the patient, he was the one consoling her and telling her that they would be OK.

His disease responded extraordinarily well to the treatments. He did not require a blood transfusion for months. We would meet visit after visit and talk about how it had already been two years since his diagnosis and his disease was still not showing any signs of progression. He had already outlived the grim prognosis as it appeared to be at the outset.

The three of us chatted at each visit, chuckled at each other's jokes and he would give me life advice since he was feeling so well that there were no symptoms to treat, no issues to handle.

One day when I walked into the room, I saw something unusual. He had not shaved in a few days. He looked like he may have lost five to ten pounds. He wasn't looking as sharp as he always did.

I looked at his blood work again thinking I may have missed something and perhaps his disease was progressing, but everything looked perfectly fine.

"Kelly didn't join you today?" I asked, noticing her conspicuous absence.

"Did you hear about the rare case of a patient dying from Eastern Equine Encephalitis last month? Apparently, it is such a rare disease that it had to be reported to the Department of Health and was all over the news," he said.

"Yes of course that case was discussed in every Grand Rounds in hospitals across the city but how were you involved with that?" I was still clueless as to why he was trying to change the topic.

"That was Kelly. My Kelly." His eyes filled with tears.

"Oh, I'm so sorry to hear that Mr. Hendricks. I'm truly very sorry!"

"I was the one who was supposed to be old and dying from terminal cancer, but here I am, doing perfectly fine and she left me. I did not see that coming."

"Neither did I." I consoled him as best as I could but felt that I couldn't, no matter what I said.

The next few appointments were difficult. Physically he was still doing miraculously well but emotionally he was being challenged.

Most of his friends had either died or were too busy in their own problems to be able to spend any time with him.

He had two children who lived out of state and because of their jobs and kids, could not take enough time off to visit him. He would not move in with them because he could not let go of his autonomy.

A handful of distant relatives lived locally but were able to see him only for a few hours each week. He did not want to meet new people and make new friends.

"That's not what is on your priority list when you are my age. People my age have their own issues and younger people don't have time," he explained. He missed Kelly and wanted to tell me her stories at each visit.

Another few months passed. This time he came up with an unexpected request. "Doc, I want to stop my treatments."

I could not hide my bewilderment. "But your treatments have been so successful, and your disease is in such excellent control? Stopping your treatment doesn't make any sense to me."

"I know but I'm not sure if I have anything left to live for anymore." He tried to make me understand. "Didn't you say that some people choose not to get these treatments in the first place? If that is considered appropriate, then why can't I stop my treatments now?" He had a valid question.

"Well, I have to make sure that you are not making this decision because of clinical depression, and it would be best if we had a psychiatric evaluation if you don't mind," I shared my concern with him.

"Of course, I would do anything you say," he replied.

I referred him to psychiatry to have him assessed and treated for depressive disorder. I received a note from the psychiatrist that after a careful and extensive mental health evaluation, it was determined that he neither had clinical depression nor a prolonged grieving disorder. He was assessed to have a perfectly normal decision-making capacity.

We stopped his treatments. His disease worsened rapidly. I met him for the last time in the cancer center to transition him to hospice care.

As he was leaving for the last time, he shook my hand. "Thank you for all you did for me. Thank you for letting me make my decision. I'm going home a happy man."

As I was signing his death certificate, I paused for a moment and thought about writing "Loneliness" under Cause of Death but then thinking that it may not go well with the department of Health, I signed the document after filling in the last line with "Myelodysplastic Syndrome."

My 5 Minute Conversation with A Suicide Hotline Expert

Sandy was sent to me by her primary care physician for evaluation of anemia. As I reviewed her chart, I explained to the medical student that the blood work showed a lifelong benign condition called alpha thalassemia trait that she was born with. It had no potential to harm her.

This would be a quick consult meaning we would have some extra time to enjoy our lunch. As I walked into the room, I caught her stifling a yawn. I looked at the clock to see if I had her wait for too long, but I was on time. She recognized the conundrum on my face. The following dialogue ensued:

Sandy: Hi Doc. I work over nights and just finished my night shift. Sorry, I'm a bit sleepy but I will hit the bed as soon as I get home from here. Hope you don't have bad news for me. Walking into the cancer center is scary. Your nurse just took my blood pressure, and it has never been this high.

Me: Well, I reviewed your blood work, and you have a benign condition that you were born with. This does not have the potential to cause any problems for you. So, you can go home and rest. What kind of work do you do?

Sandy: I'm a social worker.

Me: What kind of a social worker?

Sandy: I have done different kinds of social work but what I'm doing currently, for the last several years, is to work with Veterans. I'm a suicide hotline agent. I'm the one on the other end of the phone when anybody calls the 1-800 suicide hotline number, now 988.

Me: That's very interesting! I have always wanted to talk to someone who works closely with actively suicidal people. In medical school, they teach us a little bit about how to handle such a situation, but I have never personally been involved. Tell me this: If I walk into a room and someone is standing up on a chair, with a rope around their neck, ready to kick the chair or standing in the window, about to jump out, I would personally panic, but how should I act in such a situation?

Sandy: Well first of all don't panic. Try to stay relaxed. Don't be afraid of starting to talk to the suicidal person. Just take it easy and say something. Talk to them about anything.

Me: That would be hard, I guess. I would be too worried that I might trigger their thoughts further.

Sandy: Yes, that's the natural way to think but just ease into the conversation. Engage them as much as you can. Ask them what's going on. Hear their story. Offer them support and help. Try to come in the way of their suicide plan. For example, if somebody has a gun to their head, just ask them to put the gun on the floor for a minute so that you can talk.

Me: Has it ever happened to you that you were on the phone and somebody killed themself?

Sandy: Yes. (*At this moment she sighed and put her head back and her eyes became moist.*) There was a veteran who used to call me for support, and I had convinced him that he had to live for Arnie who was his dog for six years. He was all he had in this world. One morning he called me and wanted to say goodbye to me. I reminded him that he had to live for Arnie, and he said, 'Ma'am, Arnie did not wake up this morning.' I did not know what to say and then I heard a muffled gunshot.

Me: That's hard!

Sandy: You don't know how much I hate fireworks.

Me: What? I love fireworks. What's wrong with that?

Sandy: I cannot tell you how many vets call me on the fourth of July. It reminds them of the bombings and killings during war. At the sound of the fireworks, their PTSD triggers. It is heart-wrenching to see grown-up men curled up in their bathtubs and crying like children. I get so mad.

Me: Wow, I never looked at fireworks that way. I never thought that fireworks could have a negative impact like that on anything.

Sandy: You know we get calls from all over the world. It is free of cost from anywhere in the world.

Me: I didn't know that! That is amazing. But what if someone is speaking a different language?

Sandy: We have instant access to interpreters of any language, just like you do when you see your patients. But the problem is that I can talk to them, but I cannot send help everywhere. We are connected to the local authorities and Police in many countries but not everywhere. Have you heard of the suicide forest in Japan?

Me: Suicide forest? What in the world is that?

Sandy: In Japan, there is a forest (Aokigahara) right next to Mount Fuji. They say that people used to abandon unwanted children and the elderly in that forest in olden times. Now it is known for people to go and commit suicide there. They do it mostly by hanging from a tree.

Me: I wonder if other countries have places like that.

Sandy: Right here in the United States, the Golden Gate Bridge in San Francisco has recorded the most number of suicides in the world! In fact, they are trying to build suicide barriers that have still not been completed after all these years.

Me: You have such a difficult job, Sandy.

Sandy: I think that you have a difficult job. I couldn't do your job. People call me when they want to die, and I try to convince them to live. People come to you when they want to live, and you have to tell them that they have to die.

Me: Well, we are all placed in this world to do the jobs that we can. Humans are resilient. Sometimes we have no choice but to adapt to the task that we have been assigned to. People often think that our jobs are depressing but some of the happiest people I have seen are those that work with death and dying. You will never see a depressed hospice nurse, funeral director, gravedigger or executioner. I guess the daily reminder of death prepares us well to accept it when it knocks on our door. And also enables us to live each day to the fullest since tomorrow is never promised.

Sandy: True that Doc!

Me: Anyways, it looks like I got more out of this clinic visit than you did! How much is the co-pay that I owe you? (*We both chuckled.*) I hope that I can use the information that you gave me some day and save somebody's life. As for your anemia, you don't need to see me again.

Donna Necci

Our first meeting

My first memory of Donna is when she came to the Cancer Center for the first time. She had been recently diagnosed with cancer that had already spread to her liver.

As I walked into the room, I found an energetic and charismatic person who had the ability to become the center of attention of any gathering.

You did not have to know Donna for a long time to see that every word that came out of her mouth came straight from her heart. There was absolutely no pretense and nothing fake about her.

I introduced myself as her oncologist and she started with a litany of complaints.

"Listen, doctor, we have our own business, and we know how to run a business, and I can tell you that you guys are not doing the best job around here. I am not getting a good feeling so far," she said.

"Thank you for bringing that to my attention. We take great pride in what we do around here. We will do what is best for you and sometimes we may tell you to do something that you may not like but we will still say that to you if we think it is in your best interest. Just like family members do for each other. When people come to your business for services, you call them customers. When people go to lawyers, they call them clients. But now you will know that when people come to doctors, we call them patients. This is because we want you to be patient in order for us to help you," I responded defensively.

As I was speaking, I saw her intently looking at me and listening to what I was saying. I could tell that she was a woman of resources and had a variety of choices in where she wanted to go to get her cancer care. I was expecting that she might get angry or upset at what I was saying and was preparing myself for more complaints from her but then she said something that took me totally by surprise.

"You know what? I have decided that you are going to be my doctor!" she declared.

Not knowing exactly how to respond, I muttered, "OK..."

"Won't you ask me why?" she asked.

"Why?"

"Because you have a bump on your ear, and I have it too!" she pointed towards her ear.

I burst into laughter and everybody in the room laughed. This was clearly not the direction that everybody was expecting the conversation to take.

"I can see that. So far other than myself, I know of only one person who has a similar bump on his ear and that is my son. In fact, my son looks very much like his mother's side of the family and the ear bump is the only way I can be assured that he is my son," I chuckled. "And now you are the only other person in my life who also has the bump!"

She had used her magic to make an instant connection with me. We had both declared to each other that we would not just be in a doctor-patient relationship but would rather operate as family members.

Little did I know that over the course of the next couple of years, she would make intimate and personal connections with literally all the staff at the cancer center.

The life that she lived with Stage IV cancer

When Donna was originally diagnosed with cancer, it had spread to her liver, but fortunately she did not have any severe symptoms. She started chemotherapy, which she tolerated very well. She kept on living her life to the fullest.

She was very social, outgoing, and flamboyant. She kept on doing all the things that she wanted to do. Nobody could tell that she was living with Stage IV cancer.

Other than myself, she was seen frequently by our nurse practitioner Maria Paddock and developed a very close personal connection with her. She was on family-like terms with all the nurses and secretaries that ever were involved in her care.

Every few days, some staff member from the cancer center would stop me in the hallway and ask how Donna was doing. They always had a concern similar to what you might have for your family member.

Our staff often gets emotionally involved with most of our patients, but I do not think that I had been asked about any patient by my staff as much as I was asked about Donna.

She was also very fond of giving gifts. Especially around the time of the holidays, she would bring personalized gifts for many of the staff members. These were not just random gifts, but you could tell that she had gotten to know each staff member on a personal basis and got them gifts that they liked.

We would tell her that she did not really need to do that, but she told her that she was doing that out of her own happiness. Even as I write this eulogy, I am sipping coffee from a mug given to me by Donna that she gave me to celebrate a marathon that I ran.

Sue Rosica is one of our deeply respected nurses who has worked with cancer patients for several decades. You would think that she may have been "hardened" by this job of taking care of cancer patients and then losing them. She told me how Donna had made a personal connection with her too at their first meeting.

Sue had seen her birthdate on her clinical chart, and they instantly connected when they found out that they were exactly the same age, only twenty days apart.

Donna found out that Sue liked gardening and brought her an Italian Rose bush that she had kept at her house that reminds her of Donna now that Donna is gone.

Sue often talked to Donna about her grandsons, and they called them the Zucchini brothers. Donna would ask about them often and they became more like friends on top of their nurse-patient relationship.

No wonder Sue's tears would not stop flowing when I saw her at Donna's funeral services.

The Auction

Donna started telling me how she was planning to host an auction event at her Lake House. "Listen, we are not the richest people around town, but we do well."

She put together an extravagant event and invited a lot of friends, many of whom were quite resourceful. She arranged for an auction with the intent to raise money for the cancer center. The outcome of the auction was very interesting.

"I was expecting to raise a few thousand dollars, but I ended up raising 36,000 dollars!" she exclaimed.

"That is a lot of money Donna. How did people end up donating so much?" I inquired.

"Well, you know me! I had them serve the alcohol first and then we started the auction when everybody was quite tipsy and then they got carried away with their donations," she replied, and we both had a good laugh.

"I am going to donate this money to the cancer center, but it will be in your name. You do whatever you want. If you want to take the nurses out on a cruise, so be it but you have to decide how this money gets used," she told me.

"Donna, you are making it very hard for me to be able to thank you for that. But I will make sure that every penny gets used where it is needed the most," I promised.

The cancer center administration was of course quite appreciative of her donation. A small ceremony took place where her generosity was highlighted and shared with the community by a local news channel.

The hospital also honored her by dedicating an office suite in our names. This was particularly honorable for me to have my name on the plaque since this kind of honor is typically achieved towards the end of one's career.

This is how Donna battled her own cancer. By giving to others and focusing on a mission to make people happy.

Mike

Nothing can ever be said about Donna without a mention of Mike. When patients come to us for their medical care, their family members also become our patients, in a way. They are the doctor's eyes and ears at home. We collaborate with them to give the best possible care to the patients at home.

If any big decisions are made, although the final decision is always the patient's, but we make sure that everybody present in the room is on the same page. Mike was always by Donna's side. He always kept such a calm demeanor.

The thing that struck me the most was how much Mike loved Donna, without uttering a single word about it. In my estimate, very few men are capable of loving a woman as much as Mike loved Donna. She would always be talking and joking, the usual charming Donna, and I could see him constantly smiling, laughing, and doting over Donna.

Mike never contradicted Donna. He always channeled her thoughts in the right direction. He did not say much but was always a great listener and asked the best questions and was there for Donna as a strong pillar and a firm anchor.

When Donna saw death, a year before her death

About two and a half years after her diagnosis. Donna was still living life about the same as she had since before her diagnosis. She tolerated chemotherapy exceptionally well and had no symptoms. As much as I was happy for her, I kept giving her subtle warnings that things might not always stay the same. Then one day, her cancer finally decided to wake up in vengeance, ending its deep slumber.

We had just had a clinic visit and discussed her latest scans, which showed that cancer was quiescent and growing at a very slow pace. We decided to change her chemotherapy regimen. This was a time when we were least expecting any problems. She was making plans to travel and have a very busy social calendar.

A few days later while she was at home, just over a matter of a few hours, she started having pain in her abdomen that started out of nowhere and kept intensifying. This escalated rapidly to a point that she had to be brought into the hospital emergently. Her bowels had been obstructed by the cancer and because of the blockage, the infection had spread into her bloodstream. She rapidly started losing her blood pressure and went into septic shock.

We routinely see patients whose bowels get obstructed and just by giving some days of bowel rest, they recover but Donna's condition was worsening every passing minute. The ICU doctors and the infectious disease experts felt that this might be a life-ending event for Donna. The surgeon had to be called in immediately as an emergency.

It was a difficult situation since her risk of dying from surgery was high, but she was still taken to the Operating Room and the skillful surgeon operated to relieve the obstruction but in doing so, had to remove a large part of her intestine.

Donna had to stay for several weeks in the hospital for recovery. Mike remained by her bedside as if someone had glued him to her hospital room.

When Donna was in the hospital, it is no exaggeration for me to say that almost every day when I went to work, someone from the cancer center would stop me in the hallway and ask how Donna was doing.

After Donna came out of her coma, I visited her. She seemed to be in a state of shock. From her eyes, you could tell that she had seen death from up close. Death had visited her and wanted to take her but decided to walk away for a while. For how long? We did not know.

Donna never fully recovered from this incident. She kept on losing weight.

Since a large part of her intestine had to be removed, she could not get enough nutrition and hydration on her own. She had to come to the cancer center multiple times every week to get fluids through her veins.

Any other person who would have such a change in their life overnight, that is, from having a busy social calendar and from going to cruises and concerts to now having to sit in the cancer center hooked up to IVs would not take it very well. But not Donna!

You could still see the sheer bravery and courage in her eyes. She kept her charm and sense of humor. She was already beloved at the cancer center but now she was also spending more time with our staff.

Our nurses are some of the best nurses in the hospital and they already take great care of their patients, but you could tell that when they were with Donna, they were treating her like their own family member and were giving her genuine love. They were only returning the love that they had already received from Donna. What you sow, so shall you reap.

Our Final Meeting

Finally, a time came when Donna's body was not even strong enough to receive any more treatments such as chemotherapy. She continued to lose weight.

In a lot of cases, patients and their family members and also the nurses wait for the doctor to declare that a patient should now go on to hospice. That no more treatments are possible and the only way to move forward would be to keep the patient comfortable and to stop any potential life-prolonging treatments because they would only add to the patient's suffering.

In Donna's case, although I was supposed to have the final word as to when to offer to initiate hospice level of care, all my experienced nurses and nurse practitioners had already made that decision for her.

In my conversations with my team, I was told by multiple experienced nurses that they thought that it was now time that Donna should stay at home or be in a hospice.

I walked into the room. Donna was seated in a recliner wrapped up with warm blankets. Mike was by her bedside as always. All that remained of her was skin and bones. Her face had the classic look of "cancer cachexia."

We had talked about this moment multiple times through the course of her illness. She realized that the time had now come for her to say her goodbyes. There was peace on her face. There was understanding and acceptance.

On one hand, I was telling her that it was time to stay at home and spend quality time with her loved ones. I asked her to call anyone close to her to have her final conversations and goodbyes. But on the other hand, I myself did not have the heart to say goodbye to her. I told her that this is not goodbye and that I will be around for any issues or concerns. I left the room with that thought.

One week later I received the department notification that she had passed.

What did we learn from Donna

Donna came into our lives and taught us several things in the process. When I went to her funeral services, all her family members came to me and thanked me for the care that she received at the cancer center. They told me that Donna loved everybody at the cancer center.

"What you put in; you get back. Donna gave nothing but love to everybody at the cancer center, so they were returning only what they had received from Donna in the first place," I said to them.

They told me that she had already arranged her funeral services and remained in control of arranging all the formalities dealing with her departure from this world. Instead of flowers, she asked people to donate to the Cancer Center.

She taught us how to remain in control of any situation even when it meant that you would lose control at one point. She taught us how to make personal connections and then follow them through. She showed us how to live a beautiful, energetic life full of experiences even when faced with the prospect of living only another few years.

A Cancer Patient's Last Wish

It's not a good feeling when as a doctor, you cannot do too much for your patient. That's how I felt when I walked into the room to see Valerie for the first time.

She was in her sixties. She was flanked by her two adult granddaughters who you could tell were very close to their grandma. You could tell that at some point in her life, when she was younger, she may have been an athletic person, but now she was reduced to skin and bones.

Valerie couldn't walk without assistance and that's why she was sitting in a wheelchair which was taking up a lot of room in the relatively small exam room.

She had certainly aged a decade more than her real age. This was reflective in the wrinkles on her face. Some wrinkles are age related but hers looked like wrinkles of self-abuse.

The kind of wrinkles that people develop when they smoke and drink a lot. I'm not even sure if there is such a thing, but we all have seen people who start looking a certain way if they abuse their bodies.

Valerie had a raspy cough clearly indicating that she had a cigarette right before entering the room and was waiting impatiently for her next one which she would smoke as soon as we were done with the visit.

I had already read in her chart that she woke up one day and her eyes looked yellow as if her grandson had colored them with his Crayola's.

Before that, she had already lost more than twenty pounds, but she was attributing it to cutting down on energy drinks. She wasn't in any pain. Yet.

Tests had shown that she had developed pancreatic cancer that had spread to her liver and lungs. Her kidneys had also taken a hit, and the nephrologist had told her that she was lucky that she did not need dialysis right away but that she may need it any time.

Food tasted like garbage. Breathing was OK but every few minutes she had a feeling that she had to catch her breath.

While her body was wilting away rapidly, her eyes were filled with hope as she was talking to me.

"Typically, we are able to give chemotherapy which doesn't cure this kind of cancer but can buy us some time and also quality of life. In your case however, I think chemotherapy will be worse than the cancer because your body is too weak to go through it," I said.

"So, what do we do then Doc?" she inquired desperately.

"We will make sure that you are comfortable, and we will focus on your symptoms. It would be best that you transition to hospice level of care," I responded.

"You mean you want me to go home and die?" she asked.

"In a way, yes. If you were my mother, I would say the same thing."

The hope in her eyes shut down just like how lights go off in a theatre after the show ends. She did not say anything for a few minutes. Her granddaughters became tearful, and I offered them tissues.

So far, whatever was happening in that room, was quite a routine occurrence for me and scenes like that are unfortunately a daily occurrence in a cancer center. But then she said something for which I was not prepared.

"Hey Doc. You remind me of my boyfriend that I had when I used to live in New York City." Her eyes went into a reminiscing dreamy state for a moment. "He was the best man that I had ever had. He left me but I never found a man like him ever again."

I became paralyzed for a moment because I did not know how to respond. I just nodded. "Thank you, I'm flattered." That was all that came to my mind to say.

"He was from Pakistan and took care of me like a man takes care of his woman." Now she was looking at me in the eye.

"I am also from Pakistan," I told her.

This was probably her way to change the topic of her grim prognosis and make the moment lighter. She wanted to be brave for her granddaughters and show them that even the news of death couldn't break her. She shook off the grief and a cute mischievous smile spread across her face. She saw me getting slightly uncomfortable in my chair and proceeded with her flirtation.

"He used to make the best lamb curry for me." Her mouth watered probably for the first time since cancer rendered her taste buds useless.

"That's interesting, because I also make lamb curry that my friends like so much, I must have made it for them dozens of times," I smiled.

"Doc, would you fulfill a dying person's last wish?" she asked, looking at her granddaughters as if to get a kick out of how she was now playing with the doctor's emotions. "I want to have Pakistani lamb curry for the last time. Will you make it for me?" she asked.

"C'mon gramma, that's not what you're here for," one of her granddaughters said embarrassingly.

Thinking to myself whether she was serious or just joking, I told her I couldn't promise anything.

We did not make any follow up appointments, and she went home on hospice level of care, or to die, in her own words. I went on seeing the rest of my patients for the day and went home.

The weekend came and no matter what I did, my mind wandered to our conversation. My mind kept telling me that she was just joking. Who does these things nowadays? Maybe she had even forgotten what she said to me.

But then how could I not fulfill her last wish? How often are you given the task to fulfill the last wish of a person?

In the legal system, in those places where a death penalty is given, isn't it a thing that that last wish of a person is asked and then fulfilled? It's as if it's the dying person's right that should be granted whenever possible.

Finally, I decided that I would make her lamb curry.

While I was cooking, I was thinking whether she would even be able to eat it due to her disease. At the time of adding spices, I thought whether I should use my usual amount of spices or cut it down? What if it's too spicy and she gets nauseated?

I looked up her address in her medical chart and took the neatly boxed lamb curry and a packet of naan.

The neighborhood was not the nicest part of town. I found her house and knocked on the door. A young woman opened the door, and we instantly recognized each other. She was one of her granddaughters. She saw the boxes of food in my hand and yelled, "Hey grandma, you wouldn't believe who's here."

I walked into the house. It was very small. There she was, sitting in the living room on a couch. She had an oxygen tube in her nostrils. She appeared a bit drugged probably from the morphine.

There were at least a dozen empty cans of beer on the table in front of her. The ashtray was full of cigarette butts and rather than emptying it, she was now using the beer cans as ashtrays.

There was a thick cloud and the smell of marijuana in the room. She was a little disoriented perhaps from all the prescription and non-prescription drugs, but she still recognized me.

"Did you really think that I would not fulfill your last wish?" I smiled and put the lamb curry in front of her and instructed her granddaughter how much time to heat it up for in the microwave.

Valerie wasn't in a condition where she could have a long conversation with me, but she knew exactly what was going on.

I saw her eyes smile for a moment that tore through the pain that was otherwise displayed all over her face.

She didn't say much, but just enough when she said, "God bless you."

I left her house wondering to myself that we have always read in books that when somebody is given the death sentence, they are asked about their last wish. We seldom do that in medicine. Should we?

To my Patient Who Will Lose Her Hair from Chemotherapy

Dear Patient, I understand that the biggest fear you have about going through chemotherapy is that you will lose your hair. I just want to tell you. You will be fine. Trust me.

I know it's barbaric. In this day and age, why don't we have medicines to treat cancer that will not make you lose your hair? Strange, right? But science has its limits.

Work is being done on finding such drugs, but we are not there yet. If you google "Forced Standing," a black and white picture of a girl from a couple of hundred years ago pops up who is being forced to stand, by tying her neck and arms with ropes to the ceiling and walls. Her head is slightly slumped over to one side as if she does not want to stand.

The caption will inform you that this is actually how clinical depression was treated at that time. The idea perhaps was that if someone is depressed and is lying in bed all day, forcing them to stand up would somehow cure depression.

When we look at that picture today, it seems like a scene out of a horror movie. Whoever I have shown that picture to, has gasped.

But at that time, this treatment was likely endorsed by some, if not all, psychiatrist societies of the world.

Human history, after all, has no deficit of theories and rituals that were popular at the time but later considered abhorrent.

Now we think that we are living a very modern life. We are proud that medicine has advanced tremendously over the last few decades. The human lifespan has doubled over the last century due to medical marvels like vaccines and antibiotics.

But we don't realize that still, some of our medical practices would be considered barbaric and horrific after a century or two.

One of them will be the fact that we had to give a drug so toxic to kill cancer cells that it would destroy normal cells too. A man of the next century will gasp similarly when shown a picture of a woman from today, bald as a result of her cancer treatment.

But describing chemotherapy like that falsifies its perception in people's minds. As of the current knowledge of human beings, it still is the best treatment out there for cancer.

Thankfully, most of the new categories of anti-cancer treatments do not cause baldness but we are still a few decades away from having these new drugs fully replace chemotherapy, but the era has already begun.

For as long as we are stuck with chemotherapy, you will have to take it. It will save your life. Yes, you will lose your hair after a few weeks. Most women tell me that they are fine for the first couple of weeks but then they start having chunks of hair coming out, typically while taking a shower.

From then on, depending on the chemotherapy regimen you're getting, it comes out fast and you are left with very thin hair with your scalp showing.

Some women, once the hair starts falling, will get their hair shaved saving themselves from the trauma of losing more hair every day. Get rid of it all at once, they say.

As your oncologist, I have to worry about dozens of very serious side effects that you can get from chemotherapy. Several of them can actually end your life before the cancer does. From that standard, losing hair does not seem to be such a big deal. You lose your hair to save your life, not a big deal.

But I am not so cruel or stone-hearted not to understand that your worries and perception are different than mine. You are not thinking about neutropenic sepsis or disabling neuropathy. You are worried about how you will look.

Will people look at you with sympathy? How will you face people? I want you to know that your worries for yourself are as important to me as my worries for you.

For how long have you had the same hairdo? Most women (and men) tell me that they have had the same hairstyle for so many years. We are so resistant to change in life. But change can be refreshing. It can be uplifting.

Look at movie stars. Look at Tom Hanks and Meryl Streep. They are always changing their looks and appear in each new movie with a new hairdo. We get so used to their different appearances that we don't even remember what their "original look" is like.

In life, we all know some people who are changing their appearances not too infrequently and we learn to mentally accept them in any of their getups.

Some women who I have seen that deal with losing hair from chemotherapy best, are always "rocking" new looks at each stage of their treatment. They either carry a bald look or use very beautiful and cool scarves and bandanas. Others use wigs that, please don't tell them, often look better on them than their own hair!

When their hair starts re-growing, they have a new way of styling any length of hair. They look beautiful at any stage of their hair loss and regrowth.

You should also know that your fear of losing hair is actually your fear of the opinion of others about you. If you were to be alone for those months that you would lose your hair, you tell me that you would be fine. You would not want to see people or go to places and rather stay at home.

I understand that can be intimidating, but I want you to identify this fear and tell yourself that the last thing you should be worried about is 'what will people say.'

This is your body; you are fighting a deadly cancer, and it is nobody's business to think or say anything about how you look.

In fact, this may just be in your head, because any person who knows and loves you and is caring for you right now, will accept you any way you look.

Think of it like when you were pregnant and had your baby. You went through several months of nausea, bloating, weight gain, and other unflattering symptoms. Your body was changing as you could never imagine. There was a point when you looked at yourself in the mirror and became tearful at your appearance.

After your baby was born, with some effort, your body went back to close to where you wanted it to be. In fact, even more beautiful than prior. You developed the glow of a new mom.

When you look at your child, you have a feeling that it was all worth the effort and you would be willing to go through a hundred more pregnancies like that to have your child.

Losing your hair with chemotherapy is similar where the reward is in the shape of a saved life.

Trust me when I say that I feel as frustrated as you do about losing your hair to chemotherapy. But this is the best I can do for you. For now.

Which one is Worse? Having Cancer or Feeling Ugly?

We first met about two years ago when she came to see me in my clinic as a new patient. I glanced through her chart and reviewed her scans and pathology reports. She had one of the worst possible kinds of lung cancers, called small cell lung cancer, that had spread to both of her lungs.

Her disease was incurable, but I could give her chemotherapy to improve her symptoms and to hopefully buy her a few more months of life.

I walked into the room and found a pleasant and poised 68-year-old woman sitting nervously with an admixture of fear and hope in her eyes.

She was a beautiful woman who was nicely dressed, and there was an air of elegance and calm about her that reminded me of my mother. I instantaneously had a feeling of affection towards her.

We spoke for about an hour, and I explained everything to her in simple language, avoiding medical jargon trying to give her the right balance of hope and realistic expectations. She listened intently and asked the usual questions to which my answers were well-rehearsed.

She then asked the ultimate question, "How long do I have, doctor?"

"Most people in your situation will have another year or two to live," I replied.

She kept a straight face and blinked her eyes carefully to suppress the tears. She reached for the tissue that I offered her trying to stifle the tremors of her hands but kept her composure.

"It is what it is!" she responded and headed to the check-out desk to make her chemotherapy appointments. I moved on to my next patient.

She tolerated chemotherapy very well and enjoyed a good quality of life for two years. She had a few symptoms here and there, but mostly she was able to live close to a normal life. Her first scan after a few months showed dramatic shrinkage of her tumor.

Scan after scan continued to look good, with her disease becoming very quiet, not showing any signs of progression.

Eventually, I stopped her chemotherapy and placed her on a less toxic medication regimen to keep the cancer at bay.

She also underwent preventative radiation to the brain, which affected her mental sharpness slightly but without any major decline in her cognitive capabilities.

Soon after, she came for a follow-up visit. She had already outlived the grim prognosis that I gave her at the outset. Her latest scans were still not showing any sign of disease progression. I walked into the room excitedly and shared the good news with her.

I was expecting a joyful moment of celebration, but to my surprise, she started crying. With a puzzled look on my face, I asked her why she was upset when the cancer was under such good control.

"Look at me, doctor, I feel so ugly. I have never looked this ugly in my entire life!" She cried. I froze in my chair.

Up until this moment, I felt that having gone through so many years of training, I had a proposed solution for all of the symptoms that my patients complained of.

But nowhere was I ever taught what to do about a patient who feels that they look ugly. I could have moved on to talk about something else, but I took it upon myself to help her overcome this symptom.

My natural initial response to her was to say, "I don't think you look ugly. You look perfectly fine to me."

She faked a smile in return, but I could see in her eyes that this run-of-the-mill consolation did nothing for her. Wanting to penetrate her mind, I took a long look at her.

She had lost her hair initially due to chemotherapy, but it had started to grow back. Her hair was gray, and she was wearing a baseball hat to hide it.

Her face had become swollen from all the steroids she had received. She had gained weight and was wearing loosely fitted clothes without any care for matching or color coordination.

"Before you had cancer, I remember you had such nice and dark hair. Have you kept it gray now on purpose?" I found myself giving hair advice to a patient my mother's age, not knowing how she would respond.

"The nurses told me I could not dye my hair while I'm going through chemotherapy, and also, I just don't care for my hair anymore," she explained.

"As your oncologist, I would like to overrule my nurses' well-intentioned recommendation and ask you to go ahead and dye your hair, not worrying about any interaction with chemotherapy," I thundered. "Style your hair just the way you want and stop wearing the baseball hat to hide it."

As a man, not very well versed in different ways how a woman can groom herself, I wanted to come up with more suggestions but felt helpless. "I don't care how you do it Jody but get your game back on!" I went on.

I was a bit nervous about how she would perceive my advice. She could find it inappropriate and report me for making personal remarks.

But I believe she sensed the sincerity in my words and appeared invigorated, uplifted, and excited. "Doctor, you will see now how I get my game on!"

She asked me when her next scans would be, and I told her, to make an appointment at the hair salon and then I would schedule her next round of scans. We struck a deal, and her body language changed. She jumped out of her chair and walked out of the room like a woman on a mission. A mission to look good. A mission to not feel ugly.

I made a mental note to myself that moving forward, as I will be ready to treat any symptoms she gets from cancer, I will also make sure that we do everything for her to feel beautiful. Just like she actually is.

A Word with Vaccine Doubters

This essay was written in 2020 when the world was in the grip of the COVID pandemic.

Can you tell the difference between an 'anti-vaxxer' and a 'vaccine-doubter'?

An anti-vaxxer will outright deny and reject vaccines and may be quite rigid in their views. In contrast, a vaccine-doubter understands the importance of vaccines but has many valid inquiries.

The latter may be more accepting of meaningful discourse, so here I am, trying to have a conversation with a vaccine-doubter.

The world is facing a pandemic that no living human being has ever personally experienced. The last pandemic was about a hundred years ago and anyone who was alive to witness it at that time is long gone by now.

Thus far, humanity was clinging to hope, and I would often hear random comments about how people were exasperated at the slow pace of developing a vaccine. Finally, now when the vaccine is available, I am surprised at how many people show reluctance about receiving it.

It is difficult to convince people to prevent an illness before it happens or to treat an asymptomatic illness. Symptoms lead to compliance with the treatment. For example, many people will not take their blood pressure or diabetes medications simply because of the lack of symptoms.

Still, they will take abundant over-the-counter pills for minor symptoms. If you have a heart attack, you or another person will call the ambulance, and within a matter of minutes, you will be wheeled into a cath lab, and a cardiologist will be opening your coronary vessel.

On the other hand, you may have a large tumor growing in your chest for months, but you will not notice it unless it becomes symptomatic.

As an oncologist, it is very routine for my patients to criticize their primary care physicians for "missing" the diagnosis until it's too late. I tell them that it is the nature of cancer because it is a silent killer.

Similarly, it is difficult to "sell" the idea of vaccination since the vaccine-doubter will think to themselves, "I feel fine! Why do I need the vaccine? Maybe I might not get the disease in the first place."

As a vaccine-doubter, you may have many questions, such as whether it is a "plot" to inject the masses to control their bodies or to change their DNA or achieve some other concocted ulterior motive.

Why doesn't that thought cross your mind when you are admitted to the hospital with shortness of breath, and the doctors are giving you antibiotics or diuretics?

That is partly because currently you are asymptomatic and have time to think, but the moment you get sick, you do not want a delay of a single moment in getting the treatment. Isn't that a form of hypocrisy?

I grew up in the northern part of Pakistan. After a peaceful childhood, I had to see my beautiful region go through turmoil due to the spillage of the conflict between the USA and the Taliban.

As a medical student, I was involved in the campaign to vaccinate children against polio, which was eradicated in the rest of the world but still an emerging threat in that region.

Doctors and nurses were putting their lives in jeopardy by knocking on each door. It was hard to convince the locals that the free-of-cost oral drops vials we brought with us were for their own good.

They brought intuitive concerns that perhaps the same "foreigners" bombing their villages were sending us with vials of poison labeled in the English language.

We, the local doctors, did our best to convince them otherwise and asked them to put their blind trust in us.

Many parents did and allowed us to administer the vaccine to their children.

A few years later, Osama Bin Laden was found and killed in the same region. It turned out that a local Pakistani doctor was a key person who gave the CIA the information that led to the successful operation.

While it was great news for the rest of the world but for the doctors of that region, it was a major blow to the trust that we had tried to build for so many years with the public.

"See! We told you that the doctors are not our well-wishers, they are with the foreigners, they speak their language and wear their clothes and now they bring their medicines to give to our children and sweet talk us into giving poison to our kids!" One parent lamented, echoing the general sentiment of feeling betrayed.

Indeed, sometimes the doctors may not always be right, but those instances are rare.

A couple of decades ago, Hemophilia patients acquired AIDS from products and blood transfusions. Initially, doctors did not know that the HIV virus was being transmitted by the products they were administering to the patients.

Many hemophilia patients carried a stigma and lost their lives because of this.

The doctors later had nothing less than symptoms of PTSD riddled with a feeling of guilt that their treatments actually were the cause of death for their patients.

There are lessons to be learned from incidents like this, but for every inadvertent adverse event like that, there are examples of hundreds and thousands of instances when new treatments were successful without any unforeseen downsides.

A scientific achievement can never have success on its own unless if it has acceptance in the social context by the masses. I think that the concerns brought forward by the vaccine-doubters cannot be dismissed as ignorance, and it is hard to convince people.

As a physician, it is not uncommon that I see a patient become indecisive and anxious about various treatment decisions facing them. I don't shy away from asking them to put their faith in me as their physician at moments like this.

There is a simple strategy that makes the decision-making relatively easier, and that is to think of each patient as your own family member and recommend to them what you would want done if they were your own mother or grandfather.

When presented this way, it usually goes very well with the patient, and a bond of trust is built, which ends up in successful care for the patient.

I would say the same thing to a vaccine-doubter. If I am being vaccinated myself as a health care worker and if I agree to vaccinate my children, please trust me that you should do the same.

One Strong Woman

"Executive Director in a high-profile company." This is what was written under Occupation in her medical chart.

I was reviewing charts of patients that were new to me to go over their medical histories and order any tests that I wanted to be done before seeing them in a couple of weeks.

I like to browse social history to get to know patients even before I meet them. Sometimes I find clues that would help me get to know them better and would be a way for me to connect with them.

Her case was a routine breast cancer case for me, and I ordered the tests that were required to be done prior to our meeting.

Two weeks later, she arrived for her appointment. I walked into the room and found a woman in her early sixties sitting alone.

It is always intriguing to see who a person is accompanied by when they come for their medical appointments. A meeting with an oncologist, especially the first one, is usually a very detailed affair.

There is so much information exchanged and so many emotions tested that most people try to bring someone with them. Sometimes "for an extra pair of ears" and other times just to be with someone while going through a most difficult time of life.

Sometimes the room is full of family members to the point that one has to bring extra chairs. These, to me, are the best kinds of visits because they ensure upfront that the patient has a lot of support.

Yes, there are a lot of questions, but it is very gratifying to answer all of them to their satisfaction. The most common is when a patient is accompanied by only one other person.

Usually, it's a significant other, a sibling or a best friend. It is uncommon for someone to come alone. It leaves one wondering whether they did not have any close people in their life who could take out time to accompany them or whether they did not think much of the appointment and were underestimating the seriousness of the situation. Maybe they are a private person and do not want to burden others with their problems.

She got up from her seat and extended her hand for me to shake. After the pleasantries, we both sat down.

She was a tall woman dressed up in a suit. The kind of suit that a business official wears. She had penetrating eyes and did not lose eye contact even for a moment during our conversation. She was carrying a notebook filled with notes and on the other hand, she had an iPad with her digital calendar pulled up suggesting that she was also tech savvy, unlike a lot of other sexagenarians.

"My name is Dr. Imran and I'm a medical oncologist. I have gone through your records in detail, and I have a good understanding of your medical history, but I would still like to begin with asking you some questions." I started with my usual line reserved for all my new patients.

We reviewed how she had found a painless lump in her right breast a few weeks ago while showering. She was surprised because she was always up to date on all her medical tests including having yearly mammograms religiously.

Her mammogram only a few months ago had not shown any problems so whatever this lump was, was either missed by the radiologist or had grown too fast. Within a couple of weeks, she had seen a breast surgeon and undergone surgery to have it removed.

"The first thing we do after cancer is diagnosed is to see how much it is spread inside the body. These are the so-called stages of cancer. Your cancer was found at an early stage and has been all removed. But a cancer can come back after a few months or years as a stage IV cancer and to prevent that we have to do additional treatments that include chemotherapy and hormonal therapy," I explained the plan and its rationale to her.

"Based on your cancer's pathology, you will need two intravenous drugs. One of them is a chemotherapy drug that will go on for three months and the other one is a special targeted biological drug that continues for a year," I elaborated.

"When do you think I need to start these treatments?" she asked.

"We should start within the next month or so," I answered.

"Can I start in September?" She seemed to be calculating her options in her mind.

"That will be too late. The latest that we have started chemotherapy is within three months after surgery. That is what is done in clinical trials. We don't know how effective chemotherapy is if it is started after a longer time period than that. It has not been studied. Many think that the window of benefit is lost by then," I replied.

"But do we know for sure that it doesn't work if started later?" Now it was her time to counter me.

"No, we don't." I kept my answer brief.

"Will I lose my hair?" she asked.

This was a very common question asked specifically by women when discussing chemotherapy.

"Not with the biological drug that I was talking about but with the chemotherapy yes, unfortunately. For the first three months, you will lose your hair but then it comes back in another few months. I know nobody wants to lose their hair and this is one of the biggest stigmas that is still attached to undergoing chemotherapy but in the big scheme of things, it is a very small price to pay for such a huge benefit. To save your life," I replied.

"What if I just do the biological drug and don't do the chemotherapy?" she asked.

"Well, I don't think that would be a good decision. We don't have any studies with the biological drug alone and we don't know how much its benefit is if used without chemotherapy. Intuitively one would think that it should work but I don't have any clinical studies to back it up with," I responded.

"Can I do just the biological therapy and not the chemotherapy? I don't think that I'm in a position where I want to lose my hair," she responded.

"I would highly suggest against that," I said.

"You don't understand doctor. I know what you are saying but my situation is different. You know society has come a long way but it's still a man's world out there. I am an Executive Director at my company. There are six directors and I'm the only woman. There has never been a female director at this company. I'm the first one on their record. How do you think I reached that level? By being weak? By being indecisive? No. I have worked hard to be here. I have been tough. I have endured emotional ups and downs and worked my ass off to be here," she spoke forcefully.

"In the corporate world, nobody is your friend. Success is your only friend. It is a cut-throat culture out there. If I do not perform at any level, I lose my credibility. I cannot afford that. There are others who are waiting for me to slip, and they would be happy to push me over to take my place. But I cannot let that happen. I am towards the end of finishing a high-stakes project that involves billions of dollars, and I have to present it to the board in three months from now. I cannot let anybody know that I have cancer and am going through chemotherapy. The minute they see me without hair, everybody will know and there is a very good chance that I will lose this project. This project is the fruit of my labor, and I cannot let someone else eat it away."

She said all that with a straight face. If she was trembling inside, she did not show it.

"I have explained to you what the national guidelines for treatment are in your situation. If you want to get a second opinion, you are more than welcome to do so but I'm fairly confident that wherever you go, you will get the same recommendation," I said. "But at the end of the day, the decision is yours. If based on your situation you think this is what you want to do, I will support you. I just wanted to make sure that you are making an informed decision." I agreed with her, and we planned to start the biological treatment as she wished for.

She did well with her treatments and finished them without any major complications and more importantly, without any hair loss. Nobody knew that she was dealing with a diagnosis of cancer.

Most people take time off of work while going through cancer treatments, but she continued to work full time and finished her project like she wanted to.

We often follow patients for a few years after the treatment of their cancer and if there are no signs of the cancer returning, we discharge them from our practice.

About five years later, after concluding her annual visit, we said our goodbyes. "Let's hope that we never see each other again," I said.

. . .

During the middle of a busy day, I got a call from the emergency room.

"I have a seventy-two-year-old female who was your patient several years ago. She has a history of breast cancer and now presents with headaches for a few weeks. Initially this was treated as migraine, but the headaches were not improving. She was at the grocery store and fell down on the floor violently shaking from head to toe. She bit her tongue and had urine incontinence. The seizure was not breaking but the emergency response team arrived just in time to secure her airway and give her medicine to break her seizure. She has been found to have multiple tumors in the brain on MRI and also multiple lesions in the bones suggesting the return of her breast cancer. She is stable now and will be admitted to the floor. I thought I would let you know." The ER attending gave me a sign out.

"OK thanks for letting me know. I will arrange for her to see me in my clinic as soon as she is further stabilized and discharged from the hospital," I said.

A few days later, Lisa was sitting across from me in the clinic room.

Despite what was going on, she was still sharply dressed. Her face appeared puffy, and she had gained about ten pounds because of a heavy dose of steroids.

She was still sharp as a tack, but she was repeating her questions suggesting a possible mild impairment of cognition because of the radiation to the brain. She was still holding her notebook in her hands and had a number of different colored pens to write and highlight with.

She was accompanied by a man who she said was someone close to her. They had never given a name to their relationship, but I could call him her significant other.

"I have reviewed your biopsy with the pathologist, but this is the same breast cancer that we treated six years ago that has returned. This time it has spread to the brain, bone and the liver. It is stage IV meaning it's incurable, but we can still do treatments that can control it for some time," I explained.

"Some time? How much time are we talking about?" she asked.

"Well, we do the same treatments for all patients with Stage IV cancer, but the response varies widely. If this was some other cancer like pancreatic cancer or gallbladder cancer, the prognosis is much easier to determine but in cases like yours, I have seen patients survive only a few months if some major complication happens but we all have cases where the treatments are so effective that patients can live for many years to come, with a good quality of life," I elaborated.

"So, you mean that if I do these treatments I could live for a few months or several years?"

"That's right."

"That's very confusing to me. I have always been a very focused and organized person. I have had a very successful life and if anyone were to ask me what my greatest strength has been, I would say that it's my discipline. I am a planner. I plan every little detail of my life and then I stick to the plan. If any plan doesn't go as I want it to, I come up with a plan B. But now you're telling me that I cannot plan anything because it is uncertain how these treatments will work and how much time I have to live."

"I'm afraid that's how it is. Cancer damages the organs of your body, but it is more sinister in the way it plays with your mind. It comes unannounced in your life. Sometimes it comes with the certainty of taking your life in a short time period but other times when it doesn't take your life, it leaves you in this state of uncertainty. It is never easy," I replied.

"But how do I plan my life in this situation? Look at my calendar. There are family events. There are road trips. I have to travel for work. I volunteer at the church. If I don't even know exactly how long I have left to live, how can I plan for anything? This is making me very anxious." She shared her worries.

"Well, I would say that now that the cancer is back with a vengeance, you will have to cut down on your activities a little bit. The goal is still for you to be able to do many things that you want to do but it might not be the same as before. Also I can tell you that I'm a planner too and I know exactly what you mean by becoming anxious if you cannot plan meticulously for anything but my advice would be for you to pencil in your plans rather than putting them down with a pen so that you can be more flexible if you are not able to follow your plans. "In a few weeks to months, if your treatments are successful, hopefully you will return to a quality of life as close to prior as possible. But if things are not going well, I will tell you. My job is to tell you about your prognosis exactly how it is and not to sugarcoat things for you."

. . .

She started her treatments and never missed an appointment. She would always show up prepared with her questions, notebook in hand and taking notes, marking dates off of her calendar. She told me that she had slowed down as much as she could in her social life.

Her symptoms were manageable, and the chemotherapy side effects were quite predictable to her by now. We were getting scans every few months to see the progress of her cancer.

With every scan results she would be ready with her pens and notebooks to write down the comparisons of dimensions of her cancer lesions down to the closest millimeters.

If there was a reduction in the size of the tumors, she would express satisfaction, but she would get very anxious if there were even a few millimeters increase in size of any of the tumors despite my reassurances that we would see some growth in the cancer from time to time.

We were discussing the latest scan.

"So it looks like the cancer did not grow at all in the liver but there are some areas in the lungs that have grown and there are also some new spots on the lung. I think it's now time to change your treatment to a different kind of chemotherapy," I said.

"You said in the beginning that I could live either for a few months or several years with this cancer. With these scan results, how do you think my prognosis changes? How much time would you give me now?" she asked.

"Lisa, we have had this discussion multiple times in the past and my answer remains the same. I still have another few different treatment options remaining for you and if they are successful, you could have several more months or years of good quality of life, but it is hard to give you an exact number. It happens only in the movies when the doctor is able to tell you exactly how long you have to live," I said.

"OK let me ask you this. If I stop all treatments, then can you say with a bit more certainty how long I have to live?" she asked.

"In the absence of any cancer directed treatments, the prognosis can be relatively easier to determine. I would say that you would not have more than three to six months to live. Based on state laws, you would qualify to be enrolled under hospice level of care if we were to stop all treatments. But I would not suggest that because your life can be prolonged by a few years with these treatments," I explained.

"Well, I may live longer but that would also mean that I would be living with uncertainty. If I stop the treatments, I will have more certainty, and I can get all my affairs in order. No matter how much I try, I'm having a hard time not knowing about the future. What good is life if I have to remain anxious and uncertain all the time. I cannot plan for anything.

If I stop these treatments, although I may have a few months or years less to live but at least I will be in control of the situation. I have already paid in advance for my funeral. I can write my obituary and leave it with my family to send to the newspaper when I die. I can distribute my assets amongst my family and be prepared to leave this world and not worry about trying to live some extra months or years filled with confusion and unpredictability," she said.

"Well, it is a difficult decision to make but at the end of the day it is your decision. If remaining in control of the situation and avoiding uncertainty is more important to you than living longer, then I can see how you can justify stopping all these treatments. We typically don't see this in our cancer clinics," I said. Most people will take any treatments available even if they are told that the chances of the treatments working are negligible. A drowning man clutches at a straw. But make sure you have thought it over and talk to some of your loved ones and people who you trust just to make sure that you are convinced that you are making the right decision."

. . .

Lisa stopped her cancer treatments despite knowing that there were another few treatments available that could extend her life but without accurate predictability. She enrolled in hospice.

She stayed at her home and instead of going to doctors' offices and emergency rooms, a hospice nurse would go to their home and give medicine to keep her comfortable and ensure that she was not suffering.

She canceled all her engagements and had all her affairs in order and waited for death to knock on her door.

I saw her one last time via video.

She had lost a significant amount of weight. Her cheeks were sunken, and her wrinkles were more pronounced but there was a calm look on her face. She seemed to be in total control of the situation. She did not complain of much during that video visit and thanked me for the care over the years.

A few weeks later, the news came that she had died peacefully at her home surrounded by her loved ones. My nurse read her obituary, and we exchanged a few words in her remembrance.

"She always knew what to do but more so, she had the strength to make difficult decisions. The cancer tried to bend her on her knees and give the reins of her life in its hands, but she did not comply. She showed cancer who was the boss. She did not want to deal with the uncertainty that cancer brings and decided to stay in charge. Boy, I have seen many patients but Lisa; she was one strong woman."

Essays by a Doctor to his Peers

Is Elon Musk right about the Future of Medicine?

"Mark my words. AI (Artificial Intelligence) is more dangerous than the nukes."
Elon Musk.

The other day, as soon as I walked in to work, already running my usual ten minutes late, I was hustling from my office to the clinic when I saw one of our physician assistants in the hallway. Otherwise known for her calm composure, it seemed odd that she was visibly distressed.

She had forgotten her laptop at home and could not find a loaner. I tried to save her day by offering her my laptop to work on.

That would mean that I would have a computer to work on in the clerical area, but I would have to see patients the whole day without having a computer in the room.

She resisted but I insisted. We both went our separate ways to move on with our days.

I had not seen patients like this in quite some time now. By "like this" I mean without having a computer in the room.

Apparently, it should not be a big deal, but I realized that a computer has now become an entity that is always a part of our patient encounters.

If you don't have a stethoscope, you can get by, but you cannot do without a computer. It's as if a third "being" is present in the room, the first two being the doctor and the patient.

We interact with patients briefly but constantly work at the computer from looking up their records, labs and scans to placing orders and scheduling instructions.

Now that there is the "secure instant chat" feature, it talks back to us all the time. Other providers are messaging us constantly and, in a way, the computer keeps demanding our attention, robbing it from the patient in the room.

It gives us alerts if there are medication interactions. It reminds us to change our passwords, prompts us to order tests and stops us from closing patient charts if certain rules are not adhered to.

This particular day, since I did not have this third "being" in the room, it was just the patient and me. I felt as if the encounter was incomplete.

I kept wondering if the patient also felt as incomplete because the patient also feels reassured when they see their medical chart on the computer. "I don't remember which medications I'm taking and what surgery I had ten years ago. It's all in the computer doc!"

The patients actually have a relationship with the computer because now they look up their records themselves and try to make sense of things. Sometimes they do a good job at it and other times they suck at it. They love it for that but if the doctor spends too much time looking at the computer instead of the patient, they start feeling slighted as a jealous lover would.

Here my mind kept telling me that since I will have to document everything in the computer and use it to place orders, I would have to hurry and end the visit with the patient if I have to stay on schedule.

Then I asked myself, "How did you see patients just a few years ago? When there were no computers in the room? Relax!" A sense of calm came over me.

I forgot about having to answer constant messages and to have to place orders or to start documenting the visit. I was about to spend more time evaluating the patient and to talk about their lives and share my own stories. I felt like the crowd had dissipated.

The atmosphere in the room changed back to the intimate doctor-patient relationship that it had been for centuries.

We talked about how many cows my patient had at her farm.

We talked about how many of them they end up eating and how many they give away.

We talked about how twenty years ago, one of my patients walked in on her daughter hanging herself in the closet. Her wound is still so fresh that she truly believes that whoever says that time is the best healer is full of crap.

We talked about how one of my patients was having a robust sex life, but the treatment of his prostate cancer had taken away from him the man that he was.

We talked about how my patient's nephew was found dead from a drug overdose. She was sad for him but happy that her children did not turn up like that.

We talked about things that the third "being" in the room, the computer that is, does not allow us to talk about because we are too busy with the computer, more than with the patient.

We also talked about how I thought medicine would be practiced in a few hundred years from now. How a patient will walk through a "booth" of some sort.

His symptoms would be heard just like Siri hears us, his clinical signs photographed and interpreted. He would be scanned from the skull all the way down to the toes with all his internal organs anatomically scrutinized.

A drop of blood taken by a painless finger prick would measure all sorts of lab tests and the computer would churn out the most adequate diagnosis and treatment options and may even inject the veins with the most precise dosage of highly effective drugs against the illness.

The genetic profile of the patients would be analyzed instantly, and mutations would be identified and edited to correction expeditiously.

Complex surgical procedures would be performed meticulously by ambidextrous robots.

Humans would rely more on these "booths" than their own clinical judgment. Just like when you tell me now to calculate 89,573 x 74,823, I would rely more on a calculator then my own computing skills.

When Elon Musk warns us about the dangers of Artificial Intelligence, he is not referring to medicine in particular but we can certainly analyze his statement in the context of the future of our profession.

Will there be a day that this computer and this booth will become more intelligent than the physician's clinical judgment? "Never!" We say.

A computer has to be programmed by a human to give the results. A computer can never supersede a human's complex clinical judgment. Well to that I would say that if you tell a human from five hundred years ago that I will fly tonight from New York to Kuala Lumpur, and that too within one night! He would laugh at us and ridicule us for wasting his time.

If computers start treating us more accurately than ourselves, we would be happy to accept that. But if they start making decisions for us, no matter how, but if it indeed happens, how will they decide when it's time to stop dialysis and go to comfort care.

How will they decide how much pain is too much and when to give narcotics and when to hold them when worried about addiction?

How will they make personal connections with the patients and share anecdotes and discuss hobbies?

How will they go to funerals and how will they shed tears together with patients and their families when nothing else could be done?

How will these computers learn to give comfort and solace to these patients?

And even if they do, will the patients accept it like they accept from us human doctors?

What if they turn against us? What if they start selecting which pregnancies to carry and others to terminate? What if they start dictating the patients' advanced directives? What if they put a monetary value on the numbers of years lived?

What if they limit the number of children we can have? What if they tell me that my child is not worth living because of her disability? What if they tell me that my grandma is occupying a bed in a hospital that is needed for a younger patient and that she will be denied any more life-prolonging treatments?

What if they tell me that it's ok to clone humans and select the "best" ones? What if they assign abortion and sexual identity choices to patients?

Some of you might say: isn't that what humans are already doing to humans? Yes. You are right. But will we accept it if anyone other than humans, in this case, artificial intelligence imposes these restrictions on us?

Tired of Zoom? Bring CME Conferences to Exotic Locations

This essay was written in 2022 in the midst of the COVID pandemic

It was not too long ago, but it seems like decades when traveling for a Continuing Medical Education (CME) conference was a routine part of being a physician as looking up articles on UpToDate or giving patients bad news. But like so many other things in life, the reality of CME conferences has changed.

Most training programs give allowance to physicians for CME conferences on a yearly basis. After training, you have to keep yourself up dated in your specialty, and ongoing learning is indispensable to any medical career.

In most hospital-employed positions, physicians get days off and financial allocation for CME. In private practices, which are dying slowly as large hospital systems are engulfing them mercilessly, allowances for CME learning are factored into clinical practice and overhead expenses.

It used to be very exciting to look forward to attending the CME conferences. Most physicians attend the annual CME conferences held by their respective professional societies. It comes with a great sense of pride and achievement if your paper gets accepted to be presented in front of an international audience.

Others will choose to go to conferences that review board exam preparation materials or other such lectures that help you bridge the gaps in areas of the knowledge base that are getting rusty.

Visiting such a professional conference is a wholesome experience. The feeling of being in a room full of experts from around the world in your chosen-for-life field is full of joy.

As they walk up to the podium and deliver their talks about cutting-edge research, the speakers are given celebrity-like respect and applause.

You get a chance to ask questions and enjoy the debates that ensue when discussing controversial grey areas. You also get a chance to "hang out" with the specialist celebrity of your choice and pick their brains about individual cases. In breaks and in the evenings, you network with colleagues from other institutions.

You attend the pharmaceutical industry expositions and marvel at the financial aspect of medical care. You also attend alumni happy hours and excursions. And you return brimming with the latest knowledge, having made new contacts and refreshed by breaking the monotony of daily clinical life.

A few years ago, it was time for me to start planning to go to a CME conference. I'd be lying to you if I didn't tell you that the pursuit of academics is not the only intent for attending such conferences.

This is also a long weekend or a couple of days off with most of the expenses paid by the employer! My mind kept coming up with questions that I was too shy to ask anybody else.

Why would you not want to go to an exotic place? Why would you not think of it as a mini vacation as well? Is it bad to think of a CME trip that way?

Am I being unprofessional? Is it that in my own eyes, I fail myself that I am using an educational opportunity, partially, to satiate my recreational desires? Not finding a clear answer and concluding that my mind was ridden with 'professional guilt', I moved on.

I was between specialties. I had finished internal medicine training and was not interested in a conference in that field. I wanted to go into hematology/oncology but had not yet been matched for a fellowship, so I did not want to start going to hematology/oncology conferences either. I opened the web browser and started searching randomly, and I stumbled upon a search engine called CME Finder.

I also found CME Cruises and CME Exotic Vacations. I couldn't help smiling to myself at the thought that I was not the only one thinking along those lines. There might be enough physicians out there who may also be looking for a two-in-one deal like me. At least enough that there are multiple search engines just for that purpose.

I started looking, and you could search by cruise type and exotic location, among other options. If you wanted a specific region, they would list the names of conferences in that area, and you could choose a conference of your interest held at your desired location.

I came across a conference at an exotic beach resort location that was about medical ethics and malpractice. This was being conducted by an institute of revered reputation.

I browsed the faculty list, and there was a very interesting combination of not only doctors but lawyers from across the country, all highly qualified and accomplished and well respected in their areas of expertise.

I patted myself on my back for the excellent selection of a conference both in the learning content and the exotic potential of the location and the fanciness of the resort.

My experience of attending the conference was even better than I expected. I learned so much about medical ethics and different approaches toward clinical cases, not only from a physician's perspective but also from the attorney's viewpoint. I realized how pigeon-holed we have all become in our respective specialties.

Gaining some knowledge in a different specialty gives a new perspective and way of thinking about your own area of expertise. I decided that

I would not rule out attending medical conferences outside of my own specialty in the future.

Then the COVID pandemic happened. All the major world events got canceled. This included all CME conferences.

Zoom became a new sensation, and like everything else, all CME conferences also were changed to virtual. We are at the two-year anniversary of the beginning of the pandemic and although a few conferences are back to being held in-person, but they are few and far between and poorly attended. Although there are hybrid versions of these conferences but looks like virtual conferences are here to stay.

Don't get me wrong. The virtual conferences are supremely convenient.

You can attend via your laptop or your cellphone. You can listen to the talks in your car on your way to work or on your lunch break while you're having a sandwich. You can watch on your own time and replay if you missed a point from a lapse in attention.

But there is no denying that the excitement and the joy of the in-person conferences are lost.

Now I go to my office and lock the door. I sit alone. I watch the screen and the monotony of one speaker after another, who is also sitting at his/her office desk, making it hard to remain attentive.

My thoughts often drift to the pictures and books on the wall behind the speaker and wonder if they are wearing suit pants or pajamas. How does their choice of background reflect on their personality? There is no applause, no spontaneous laughter, or exclamations.

Between two talks, I might get up to get a coffee and use the restroom, but there is no one to talk to or share the excitement of a new point that I have learned. It is hard enough to sit through a few hours of continuous zoom talks, let alone several consecutive days of back-to-back lectures.

I hope that as the pandemic recedes, professional organizations put extra effort into conducting these CME conferences in-person again. I hope that virtual conferences do not become the new norm.

There is already talk about employers cutting down on the number of CME days allowances and financial reimbursement for airfare and lodging.

Why take a few days off to travel to listen to some talks when you can do it on your own time and from the comfort of your office chair, they say.

Classical medicine has already lost a lot of its charm by miring doctors into the web of incessant maintenance requirements of the electronic health record, which like laundry, never ends.

Ending in-person conferences will be another nail in the coffin of the joys that used to be associated with this beloved profession of ours.

Tom The Social Worker

I cannot claim to be someone who knew Tom most closely, but I can claim to be a person who asked Tom's permission to write a few words about him a few days before he died. To which he agreed.

Also, to call him a Social Worker would be a disservice to have as a title for his eulogy because he was a man of not one, but many identities and achievements. Being an outstanding Social Worker was only one of them. But that is how I knew him and will always remember him.

At the Cancer Center, before Tom entered our lives, we were already blessed to have a Social Worker, who had dedicated her life to helping patients.

She was the kind of person who lived the most fulfilling life and whose achievements both at work and home were tremendous. She, unfortunately, was diagnosed with cancer.

Imagine, helping people dealing with cancer all your life and now being afflicted with the same horrible illness yourself. She was a very private person, and we all gave her the space that she asked for. She eventually passed away amidst the tears of all employees of the Cancer Center.

The mood was low, and it was a given in our minds that there would be no way that her shoes as a Social Worker could be filled by anyone.

Working at the Cancer Center, we kind of get used to bearing loss on a daily basis but learn to celebrate the lives lost, so we did the same at her demise.

I remember when Tom joined the Cancer Center. On a busy day at work, I usually move from patient room to room and try not to stop and socialize with colleagues, otherwise, I can never get my work done. I leave that to a "slow" day. This particular day that I can recall was quite a busy one.

I was walking in the hallway trying to avoid conversation with anyone. Michele, our practice manager, walked in along with a new face who I had never seen before.

"Dr. Imran, please meet Tom. He is one of our new Social Workers." I stopped and hurriedly said hello to Tom. This is when Tom used his magic on me for the first time.

He greeted me well and engaged me in conversation in such a delightful and insightful manner, that I forgot about my busy day and stood in the hallway and spoke to him as if I had met a long-forgotten friend from high school and we had to catch up on our entire lives since we last saw each other.

Tom would often stop at my office or meet in the break room and effortlessly strike warm and friendly conversations. It is very hard to get to know another person deeply by just office small talk.

But Tom had a way of being so open about himself and such a genuine manner that I felt that I knew Tom for a very long time. He told me how his life in the past was full of mistakes. He admitted to me that for a long time, he did not fulfill his obligations in life.

He had lived a troubled past where his relationship with his family had suffered and had been badly damaged. He gave way too much to indulgence and led anything but a disciplined life, at that time. But he was proud that he had turned his life around.

He talked about that phase of life as a thing of the past. He spoke like a new person who had already conquered and defeated the old person that he was.

One of the things that connected us instantly was our interest in heavy metal music. He told me that at one time he had very long hair and all he would do was chase metal music bands. He had gone to Aerosmith concerts at least two dozen times. He told me that he once went to a local bar and there was a small unknown band playing and he thought they were pretty good.

A few years later, that same band made it into the mainstream music scene and called themselves Guns N' Roses. He had hung out with Axl Rose not thinking too much of him at that time.

I told him my story of how I love music and for a person who grew up in Pakistan, I had more exposure to American heavy metal music than many others, thanks to my uncle who used to live in Florida and would bring us cassette tapes that he recorded from FM radio.

Tom very quickly made excellent relationships with the Cancer Center patients as well as his colleagues.

We started relying on him a lot. He was the kind of Social Worker who would just take care of things. He would go out of his way to go and meet the patients and work his magic to get to know them personally and deeply. He became the usual name for our Cancer Center. "Just call Tom and he will know what to do."

One day, Trudy our nurse, walked in with a sense of urgency, "Do you think you can look at Tom's scans? He hasn't been feeling well and just got the scans ordered by his doctor. Can you or one of our physicians look into it?"

I explained the need of establishing a patient-doctor relationship with Tom's permission before anyone of us could review his medical data.

My friend Mehul (Dr. Patel) at our office took on the task of becoming Tom's oncologist. His scans had unfortunately shown that he had developed pancreatic cancer that had gone to his liver, and he now had stage IV disease which could not be cured, and he had only another year or two to live.

In life, people react differently when they are encountered with tragic events. These are the moments that define the true version of any man.

Some deal with a fighting spirit, others deal with rationalization or stoicism. Some cower and become anxious. Others remain angry or in denial.

When Tom was encountered with this situation, he dealt with it in the best way it could possibly be handled. He accepted the reality of the diagnosis but kept living his life as productive and joyful as he could. He continued to work through the illness and chemotherapy sessions.

Nobody could tell that this man, who was holding the hands of these patients dying from the same illness, helping them in any way possible, and providing them emotional support was going through the exact same himself!

During the summers, I realized that there were a lot of nice music bands who were planning to tour our area. I bought concert tickets to Billy Joel, Motley Crue, Poison, and Kiss for the summer.

Tom told me that he had already bought those tickets as well and he was planning to go with his wife Cindy. We would talk about the bands and their music and enjoy each other's love for music. Then COVID hit and all the concerts got canceled.

We were given the option of either canceling our tickets or keeping them because if we kept them, we would get better seats at the concerts when they would finally take place.

I thought that this was just a gimmick to have people hang on to their tickets instead of asking for refunds and I went ahead and canceled all my tickets.

When I asked Tom, he had kept all his tickets. His argument was that when the concerts would re-open, due to space limitations, the tickets may be much harder to acquire.

I felt guilty thinking that I should ask him to return his tickets because his prognosis from his cancer was quite limited and deep inside, I knew that he would not be able to go to these concerts because he may not be with us anymore. But of course, I could not dare to say this to him.

It's not that he did not know but he chose to ignore the fact that he was dying and rather take the positive and optimistic view of having tickets to concerts that he one day would be able to attend.

Tom kept working full time at the Cancer Center without showing any hint of appearing ill. We were all very sensitive about the privacy of his diagnosis. Whenever we used to ask him to see one of the patients, we would make sure not to tell the patients that he was facing the same catastrophe. But he was a very open and forthcoming person.

He would self-disclose to his patients and build such close bonds with them that they truly believed that they were in the same boat together and felt supported and encouraged by his demeanor.

He did not talk about retiring or having any difficulty dealing with the patients who were going through the same mental and physical agony as himself.

It was as if a ship was sinking, and everyone aboard was panicking about the imminent death, but this one person was so strong emotionally that he took it upon himself to give help and comfort to others without worrying about his own fate.

He decided to spend his last few months of life not by becoming a sorry figure but by being a hero who would be of help to others until his dying day.

This was the time that I learned the most important lesson from Tom. I would keep thinking to myself: Look at this man. He had a troubled past and he self-admittedly had problems with drugs and alcohol but then had the discipline and courage to turn around his life and dedicated it to helping people.

After doing all this, now at such a young age, he has to face a terminal diagnosis. How upset he must be with God! How he must be complaining to God that it is so unfair to him that he started doing all the right things in life but still felt punished by having such a diagnosis at such a young age.

Although I did not verbalize any of my thoughts to him, I felt that he knew what I was thinking. He proved by his behavior and his demeanor how wrong I was. He gave the air of a person who was still very thankful to God. He was not bitter at all.

Tom appeared to be a person who was happy with whatever God had written into the book of his destiny and he would accept any fate without dissent.

He often expressed gratitude that he was given a chance in life to overcome his shortcomings and eventually help others and repair all of the broken relationships he had in his previous life.

As the months passed, he started losing weight. He started having pain that was difficult to control with medications alone, so he had to go through radiation.

He would always give me an update about his health status and never said anything pessimistic or negative. I didn't even have the heart to sympathize with him because he did not appear to be a person who needed any.

Some of our co-workers started thinking about having a get-together in his honor. He had recently won a city-wide award for being the best Social Worker in town which he received at an extravagant ceremony, but we wanted to do something more intimate for him where only the Cancer Center employees would be invited.

Word went around that since he liked the music so much, we would arrange for a local band to come to our event and play some of his favorite rock songs.

Unfortunately, the COVID pandemic hit around this time and our plans could not come to fruition. This is when I had an idea! I thought that I would contact Aerosmith, yes, the actual band Aerosmith and try to write something catchy to them asking them to honor Tom as one of their top fans.

I sent a private message on Instagram to the official Aerosmith account hoping for an answer. Although this plan was not successful, I later told Tom about it, and he had a good chuckle.

This is what I wrote to Aerosmith:

"Dear Steve, Tom, Joey, Brad, Joe, Buck: I am an oncologist practicing in Rochester New York and one of my colleagues who is a Social Worker has been to your concerts at least thirty times and he is a die-hard fan. He is a recovered alcoholic and once he made his life clean, he got diagnosed with pancreatic cancer and now he is going on hospice, and he has only a few more weeks left to live. I know you have millions of fans, but I thought that I would send you this message. Who knows, maybe one of you could do something to recognize him and we will be sending one happy man to heaven. I know it's CRAZY for me to send this message but it's a SWEET EMOTION. This guy has been LIVING ON THE EDGE but then got his life BACK IN THE SADDLE AGAIN and CAME TOGETHER and now I'm DREAMING ON that you guys will recognize him in some way and that would be AMAZING." (For those who are not familiar with Aerosmith, the words in upper case alphabet are names of some of their greatest hits.)

Finally, one day I heard that Tom had decided not to come to work anymore.

He had made this decision because he had become too weak and was in a lot of pain. He had only a few more weeks left. He accepted hospice level of care which meant that he would stay at home and if he got acutely sick, he would not be brought to the hospital. A hospice nurse would visit him to provide care at his home until he would die peacefully in the comfort of his own home.

I texted him to ask him if I could visit him and he agreed. I went to his house realizing that he lived in a neighborhood by which I had passed at least a hundred times in the last few years.

Thinking to myself how we wait for someone to have a tragedy in their life to visit them rather than doing that during good times, I knocked on the door.

His wife Cindy opened the door and let me in. There he was, sitting on a couch in his living room. He appeared calm and well tucked-in in a nice blanket. His surroundings were very peaceful and comfortable. He was weak and did not have the same energy that I was used to seeing. I could not help but sense the feeling of looming death in the room.

Despite that, I could not detect even the slightest of negative emotion such as sorrow, guilt, or despair on his face.

His body was reduced to skin and bones but all I could see was contentment, closure, and a look of "been there, done that" on his face.

We spoke for about half an hour, and he made me feel as if it was any other day at work when we would stop in the hallway for an interesting conversation.

A young man appeared from another room and Tom introduced us to each other. He was Tom's son, and they had been estranged for many years but later in life when Tom got his life back on track, he reached out to his son and made amends.

He drove all the way from Adirondacks, where he lived, to be with Tom in his final few days. This was yet another sign of how Tom had repaired all the broken relationships from his past life. Tom often spoke about Cindy and his words were always filled with respect and love for her.

This is when I mentioned to Tom how I had started writing a blog and asked his permission that if someday, I wrote about him, whether it would be OK with him.

He looked at me for a moment and then nodded and as if he understood that I was looking for more affirmation, he told me that he would be fine with me telling his story. In fact, I got the feeling that he wanted his story to be told.

Tom finally left us. He showed with such class that some people, when they leave us physically, actually get even closer to us emotionally.

He taught me so much in the little time that we had together as friends and colleagues.

He taught me that if life is not going well, you can turn it around and repair it.

He taught me that if you have gone through bad times, a great way of recovering is to find people who are going through similar bad times and help them get through.

He taught me the value of stopping during a busy day and having small talk.

He taught me that it is OK to share your grief and personal suffering with others.

He taught me that if you are given the death sentence by your destiny, live each remaining day as if death was not even an issue and should not be a hurdle in the way of continuing to help others. In a nutshell, he taught me how to live, and how to die.

A Medical Student's Guide to Taking a Social History

Dear medical student (or a student in any other field that requires public dealing):

I was in your shoes twenty years ago. At that time, I thought that becoming a doctor was all about gaining medical knowledge. When I started my clinical rotations, I was convinced that the "history of present illness" is the most important aspect of patient evaluation.

As a resident, I felt that navigating through the differential diagnosis and treatment options is all that medicine is about.

Now, having been an Attending (a teaching and supervising physician) for several years, I have come to realize that it is the often ignored and underestimated art of obtaining a social history that will enable you to treat the patient rather than the disease.

You made it to medical school, so I'm not worried about your knowledge-building skills. I'm sure you will be up to date on the latest clinical trials and well versed in pathophysiology at the molecular level.

But that is all about the science of medicine and has very little to do with the art of medicine.

You will need to learn how to make personal connections with each one of your patients. You will need to build skills for the patient to like you and trust you. There is no better time to make that connection than when you are taking the social history.

No matter where your encounter with the patient takes place, be it in the emergency room or the outpatient clinic; Hospital room, or the ICU bed, you will seldom have ample time. You will often be in a rush but mind you. Social history should be the last element of your conversation that should be curtailed.

In the days of the EMR, everybody who has seen the patient before you has documented extensively so you already have a good idea about what's going on.

You probably already have a differential diagnosis in mind and are narrowing down treatment options. You can now easily spend some time getting to know your patient.

Pull up a chair and sit down, for God's sake. You will hear this a million times during your career that you should be seated while talking to a patient, but you will make mental excuses to convince yourself that you do not have enough time to sit down. You do. It's worth it.

How would you feel if you went to somebody's house, and they talked to you standing in their doorway and they don't invite you to come in and sit down? You will feel unwelcome as if they want you to leave as soon as the conversation is over.

Please don't be discourteous to your patients. If there is no chair, walk away, go to another room and bring a chair and sit down. Ask their permission and sit at the edge of their bed. I promise you that it will take less than a minute.

If you remain seated and relaxed, in the patient's perception, you will have spent twice the amount of time with them compared to the actual time spent.

As you start the encounter, it is crucial not to ignore any friends or family members accompanying your patient. Please say hi to everyone in the room and try to ask their names and relation to your patient.

If you win their hearts, these are the people who will say "what a nice doctor" as soon as you leave the room. Even if one of them doesn't like you, in case you ignored them, they will start casting doubts on your personality and judgment. Plus, it's just plain rude not to acknowledge someone in the room.

After you have asked all your medical questions, now is the time to get to the social history. Please do not start asking about their smoking, alcohol, and recreational drug interests bluntly like a robot as if you have to check off some boxes. You can do better than that.

Think of yourself at a cocktail party, and you have been introduced to someone for the first time who you are trying to get to know and want to see again. Be charming, please.

This is not just a job. This is a sacred moment where you are laying the foundation of a long-term relationship between a doctor and a patient.

Don't just ask them what they do for a living: Ask them if they like it and why?

Don't just ask them how many kids they have but ask their ages and which schools they go to.

Don't just ask them what their hobbies are, try to find common interests and give each other tips.

Don't just ask them if they are planning a vacation; ask them where they are going and with whom.

Try to remove the barrier of indifference that stands between the patient and the person that they are. I promise you they will be more than happy to answer them for you.

When you get them talking, now is the time to throw in some self-disclosure. Don't be afraid to tell them about yourself. They will love to hear from you about who you are behind the persona of the doctor.

Tell them how many kids or nephews you have and what their names are. Tell them about your hobbies. Tell them your interests outside of medicine. I know that you might not be comfortable opening up much about yourself but try it. You may find it surprising that you will win their hearts by opening up to them.

Write down some key points from what you learned about your patient in your "sticky note" in the EMR, and next time whenever you see the patient, carry on the conversation from where you left off.

Each ensuing meeting with the patient, learn more about your patient and they will learn more about you, and I promise you that within a few meetings, both of you will know each other more than you know many other people in your life.

This will make the patient trust you, and you will enjoy your job and not burn out from otherwise repetitive bland patient encounters.

When you present the case to your attending or your colleagues, start with the social history instead of the chief complaint and then see the magic.

Not only will everybody think that you know your patients at a personal level, but you will catch their attention, and they will be more likely to listen to your presentation in its entirety. Thank me after you get an excellent evaluation towards the end of your rotation.

Start doing this now, and it will become second nature to you. Learning this skill is more important than memorizing medicine textbooks.

Between you and me, it is not uncommon to see even professors, who may be extensively published and otherwise highly accomplished in their careers but would not have developed the skill to engage with their patients.

They may have the title of a professor bestowed upon them by their departments, but they will have failed miserably at winning their patients' hearts.

A Nurse is to a Patient what a Mother is to a Child

I was on inpatient service and had already seen most of the patients on my list. I just had to see one more before I could call it a day and rush out just in time to take my daughter to her tennis lesson.

I reviewed the patient's chart to find out that her cancer had spread to her spine, which had incapacitated her to the point that she could not walk on her own and required assistance even for as little as propping herself up in the bed.

I knocked on the door, but there was no response. I walked in and saw her lying in bed, trying to avoid eye contact with me.

I began to say, "Hi, my name is Dr. …" I couldn't finish the introduction because a strong stench entered my nostrils, giving me pause. The crisp white bed sheets were covered with her feces. There was a Styrofoam glass in her right hand that was also covered with feces. "I'm sorry I was thirsty!" She said in a trembling voice with her eyes filled with embarrassment.

"Don't worry, let me ask someone to help you right away," I said, trying to fill my tone with empathy rather than judgment.

I walked out of the room, headed right to the nursing station, and explained the situation to her nurse. She appeared swamped with work and busy charting in the computer but sprang up instantly and rushed to the room and, on her way, recruited two fellow nurses to help with the task.

I returned to the patient's room after ten minutes, and she was all freshened up, dressed in a fresh hospital gown, new linen, a pot of flowers, and a bowl of fruit on the table at her bedside with the TV remote and the call bell within her hand's reach.

I asked myself: Can I ever do for a patient what a nurse does? Never! Then why is it that the role of a nurse is so underrecognized and invisible as compared to a doctor's?

Ever since I wanted to become a doctor, I wanted to build long-term relationships with my patients and their families.

My dad was a pediatrician, and I used to love it when people came up to him randomly to say hi and thanks because he took care of their kids. I love it when a patient tells everyone that they are my patient and want me to be part of any decision they make.

As a doctor, I get this recognition every day, but my question is that if I had become a nurse, would I be given the same recognition even though I would have taken care of my patient with as much compassion and more "hands-on" care?

Nurses are respected but are given nowhere near as much credit as doctors.

In my mind, if the hospitals were households and all the patients were children, the value of doctors would be similar to that of fathers, and the value of nurses would be akin to that of mothers.

Fathers have their own role, which is indispensable, but it is still dwarfed compared to what a mother's role is for a child.

The roles of mothers and fathers have blended quite a bit in the modern world, but there is no denying that up until a few decades ago and still in a major part of the world, the roles are well defined.

The traditional "stay-at-home-mom" gives up everything primarily to nurture her children. She wakes them up, makes sure that they brush their teeth, wear nicely ironed and beautiful clothes, feeds them breakfast, sends them to school with a packed lunch, makes sure they are playing with their friends and doing their homework, teaches them manners on the dinner table and tucks them into bed well in time to be ready and prepared for the next day.

The "working mom" is doing all of this and on top of that is earning a living as well. Having a job gives you recognition in the form of diplomas and paychecks, but the childrearing and housework are often invisible, which becomes apparent only if it is not done.

For example, if you see a healthy and happy child, you will seldom marvel at the great job a mom is doing, but if you see a neglected child, you will instantly point towards the inadequacies of the mother.

Similarly, at the hospital, the nurse is the one who is at the patient's bedside around the clock. When the patient has to go to the bathroom or needs help to sit up in a chair, he or she calls the nurse.

The nurse is the one who is changing the diapers for the elderly; she is the one cleaning the sputum and the spilled urine; she is the one holding the patient's hand and stroking his hair while he is having a painful procedure done.

She is the one arranging the flowers and picture frames in the room. She is the one administering the medications when the patient is in pain or nauseous. She is the foremost advocate for the patient. She is at the bedside when the patient is taking his last breath, and she is the one to call the doctor to pronounce him dead after having first witnessed and confirmed it herself.

But yet, the doctor takes most of the credit. Why is that? Just because the doctor spent more years training and passed some more difficult exams and gets a bigger paycheck?

Fine, the doctor is making some of the "big decisions" in a patient's journey, but the nurse is the one who is holding the patient's hand and delivering the bedside hands-on care so selflessly.

When a patient is asked whose patient they are, they will always take the doctor's name.

I wish to see a day when they take the nurse's name as a response to that question.

When I ask my nurse to see a patient, she says, "Hi, my name is Nancy. I am Dr. Imran's nurse."

I hope to see a day when I say, "Hi, my name is Dr. Imran. I'm the doctor working with your nurse."

Also, as the gender roles in society are increasingly blending, we have not yet seen that change when it comes to the noble profession of nursing.

A few decades ago, most of the doctors were males, but now by many estimates, half are males and the other half females. I hope to see more males becoming nurses where only one out of ten nurses are a male.

A Smartphone User's Thumb

Until about 50 to 100 years ago, the tradition was to name diseases after the doctors who used to describe them for the first time. Such diseases are called eponymous diseases. There are numerous examples, such as Alzheimer's disease, Marfan's syndrome, and Wilson's disease, to name a few.

Often, specific signs and symptoms were named after certain occupations, sports or other traits.

For example, Athlete's Foot is a fungal infection of the area between the toes that often happens to active people such as athletes. Tennis elbow is pain that can develop in the elbow after performing any repetitive activity but originally associated with playing tennis. (When I got tennis elbow, my brother often joked that is when he realized that you don't have to know how to play tennis to develop the elbow!)

Achilles tendonitis is named as such because, in Greek mythology, Achilles' mother dipped him into the holy river holding him upside down and rendered him invulnerable. Only the heel was spared because the water did not touch it. Eventually, a poison laden arrow hit him in the heel leading to his death.

A gamekeeper's thumb is named as such because, in Scotland, hunters used to kill animals such as rabbits by breaking their necks between the thumb and index finger, consequently developing pain in the thumb.

Jock itch is a term used to describe a fungal infection of the groin that happens to a jock (athlete), especially when wearing a tight-fitting jockstrap, which is a type of sports underwear.

With time, the tradition changed. Now, new medical discoveries are named such that the name in itself describes the actual physical findings of a disease and is typically not named after the person who describes it. For example, Sweet's syndrome named after Dr. Sweet is now called neutrophilic dermatosis, and the list of such examples is long.

The 1918 flu pandemic is most commonly called the Spanish flu. Naturally, one would assume that the flu likely started in Spain. But this is not true.

It turns out that Spain remained fairly neutral during World War I. As a result, the media coverage was relatively free to report the actual facts and did not have to go through censorship as strictly as some of the other countries that were actively involved with war propaganda.

Therefore, most people learned about the pandemic through Spanish newspapers and assumed that it must have originated from Spain.

The COVID-19 pandemic was intentionally not named the Wuhan disease despite reports of the first major outbreak, which would bring a bad name and stigma to the place for centuries to come.

Donald Trump still made attempts to call it the Chinese virus. I'm not sure if doing so can serve any beneficial purpose.

The virus is from a family of viruses called the coronavirus family that means "crown-like" because that is what the virus looks like under a special microscope – having crown-like projections. COVID-19 is the name of the disease that the virus causes, an abbreviation for coronavirus disease 2019.

Other than bringing the world to a stand-still, the pandemic has also served to place a "seal of approval" upon the digital revolution of the last decade. The world was already going through the exponential growth of life being taken over by digital means.

However, with every new invention, there is criticism despite growth and convenience. I can easily imagine that when the microwave oven was new, people would have been reluctant to warm their food in it worrying about "rays" or other unknown ill effects.

When the car navigational system was new, people would say that if you use the GPS, you cannot "learn" your way in a new town, which was considered to be an inadequacy.

Similarly, although everybody uses smartphones ubiquitously in their lives, you can see criticism of their use and how it has changed how we interact and perhaps destroy physical relationships. Nevertheless, there always has to be a balance between innovation and tradition.

One should always be open to innovation and embrace it readily while keeping an effort to revive tradition until innovation becomes the new tradition. Smartphones and various digital formats have helped us endure this pandemic in ways that would not have been possible.

Doctors are seeing patients online, shopping is being done without going to grocery stores, banking is at the tips of our fingers, concerts and family gatherings and book clubs are taking place in cyberspace, and life is getting by. The "hands-on" jobs are still suffering but perhaps not as bad as if there were no digital means.

I am a physician, and in the last few days, I have developed pain in the outer side of my thumb. I was scratching my head to think about what physical activity I might have done that is giving me this symptom. It occurred to me that I have been using my smartphone for several hours every day, which is the reason why I have developed this annoying pain.

Now if this was a hundred years ago, I would have made an attempt at naming this symptom after myself and would have tried to publish it as Farhan's thumb, but I will stick to the contemporary practice of naming it after the cause or description of the illness — and it can thus be called "the smartphone user's thumb."

The Physical Exam is Dead

"You forgot your stethoscope!" The medical student dutifully pointed out as we were on our way to the patient room.

"I don't need it. But let me grab it anyway to pretend. But don't tell anyone I said that!" I replied. Her eyes widened with disbelief at the blasphemous statement.

At the turn of the millennium, the world was already going through seismic changes in how it conducts itself thanks to the digital revolution. Several age-old occupations were rendered redundant by automation, and new jobs were created due to innovation. Then the pandemic happened.

Social distancing stamped the new way of life with a seal of approval. Professions that were considered to be immune to any change, including Medicine, are now facing unprecedented variations in how they are practiced.

One of the first lessons taught in medical school is that the treatment of a patient is dependent on the three pillars of assessment, which include the history taking, physical examination, and the investigations, which include both laboratory and radiographic tests.

Since ancient times, medical evaluation entirely consisted of "history-taking" and "physical-examination." The inventions of the microscope in the sixteenth century and the X-ray in the nineteenth century revolutionized the world of investigation, which led to a proportional decline in the utility of the physical exam. History-taking stood its ground because even today, it is a widely accepted notion that a good clinician can solve the majority of medical conundrums just by interviewing a patient.

The physical exam consists of four parts. "Inspection" simply means looking at a certain part or the whole body. "Palpation" consists of touching a part of the body with the hands. "Percussion" is the act of placing a hand or a finger on a part of the body and tapping it with the other hand to assess the underlying area based on the type of sound it makes. This seems to be an archaic practice now. "Auscultation" is the act of using a stethoscope to listen to the internal sounds of the body.

While the physical exam still remains irreplaceable in emergency situations, it has been replaced by radiography for most of the non-urgent clinical situations.

Think of it this way; if you already have an accurate account of the internal organs down to the minute details in the form of an MRI or a CT scan, even the best of physical exams pales in comparison.

With a bedside ultrasound, you can see the entire liver or spleen and know the size down to the exact centimeters. The guesswork is gone when it comes to detecting and interpreting heart murmurs since an echo readily shows clear pictures of the heart.

As a medical oncologist, I have to routinely assess the size of tumors to know whether they are growing or shrinking, which is accurately done with scans. The neurological exam is most intriguing when a clinician is trying to "localize" the part of the brain that has a lesion, but this practice also seems unnecessary when you have a brain MRI pulled up on your screen.

Of course, this does not hold true for an emergency situation, but these tests are now done so rapidly especially for patients in emergency rooms and intensive care units that it is usually a matter of minutes when you can have a scan done and a trained radiologist giving a detailed report of the internal organs.

Why, then, are we still doing physical exams? There are multiple reasons.

The act of the physical exam is tied in with the identity of a physician. It has been such an indispensable pillar of medical practice that many physicians would consider it sacrilege to call it redundant. A stethoscope is as much the identity of a physician as it is a tool for evaluation. I have had older patients reprimand me for not giving them a thorough check-up if I have done a relatively brief physical exam. There is a certain comfort in the physician's touch where a patient develops a kindred regard for the physician.

The other major reason why physical exams are still expected to be done is the way medical visits are billed and paid for. The documentation in order to be considered billable, has to comprise of the three major elements, including the history of the illness, the physical exam, and the medical decision making. Physicians now have templates of normal physical exam documentation, which they simply edit to reflect the abnormal exam findings.

Sometimes it feels even absurd to perform all the physical exam items. Imagine having a patient who is already tearful and numb after hearing of a new diagnosis of life-limiting pancreatic cancer and despite the availability of scans showing details internal organs, it would be fairly odd at that moment to assess if the trachea is midline or to be asking the patient to perform the finger-to-nose test to assess cerebellar function.

COVID-19 served as one of the final few nails in the coffin of the ubiquity of the physical exam. Medical visits very quickly transformed from "in-person" to "virtual." This is running very smoothly, and patients are getting most of the medical care that they require. In a small number of situations, when a physical exam has to be done, patients are asked to come to the office. Patients find it very convenient to see their doctor from the comfort of their living rooms and not having to worry about transportation, traffic, parking, or the weather.

Telemedicine has been around for many years now, but it by no means was widely implemented. After COVID-19, it looks like it is here to stay. As this becomes the new norm, all the major elements of the medical evaluation will still stay the same but the previously mandatory physical exam, although still will retain its value under certain circumstances but in a broad sense, will transition from a tenet of medical evaluation to a dispensable and even archaic practice.

Essays by an Immigrant

What are your Dog's Pronouns?

There were times when Latin or Sanskrit were the most widely spoken languages around the world. Today, that claim goes to the English language.

When I was growing up in Pakistan, we used to speak Urdu and Pashto at home but since the country was under British colonial rule prior to gaining independence, English was the language that was taught in school and was considered a sign of literacy.

I can still remember that in our English grammar books in first grade, there was a chapter on pronouns. We learned that you use "he and him" for male and "she and her" for female. "They and them" were used for multiple people or objects regardless of their gender.

But I also remember that the pronoun taught to us to be used for an animal such as a dog or a cat was "it." The same pronoun was used for inanimate objects too. This was as clear to me as all the other pronouns, and I may have used "it" for animals hundreds of times without even giving it an extra thought.

After moving to America, for the first time I got to experience English as the first language. Having formally learned the English language in school and being very familiar with the American accent from Hollywood movies, I felt entirely comfortable speaking this language in my daily life.

Some immigrant friends felt the need to acquire an "American accent" and tried hard to sound American, but I never understood the significance of striving to do so since I believe that your accent should reflect where you are born and raised regardless of the language that you are speaking.

Other than language differences, there were a lot of aspects of life that were different between the two countries. One thing was the attitude towards pets in general and dogs in particular.

In Pakistan, very few households have dogs as pets. Even if there is a dog in the house, it is kept outdoors since there is a general religious perception that a dog is "unclean" and if you have touched a dog, you cannot pray. It is generally believed that a dog should only be kept as a pet either for watchkeeping or hunting but not for any other reason.

My grandfather had two dogs, Leo, a handsome German Shepherd and Doozer, a cute Cocker Spaniel. They used to live outdoors and most other people in the household rarely had any physical contact with them.

If by chance, any of them got even close to my mom or aunt, they would start panicking and rush to go and take a shower and a change of clothes to "cleanse" themselves before it was time for the next prayer.

The situation I found was completely different in America. Dogs are considered to be family members and given as much love and care as children if not more. Dogs live indoors and use the same couches and beds as other family members.

Dogs in America get better medical care than most humans in poor countries do and eat better quality food than a majority of the indigent human population in the world. They have rights and prerogatives. Their feelings and emotions matter. Their birthdays are celebrated, and their deaths are lamented. Even the "bumper sticker family" on cars includes them right next to children. Dog owners are called dog moms or dog dads.

A couple of years ago, I received a work-related email from a colleague. Under his signature was an additional line that just said, "him/his/he." I had never seen pronouns listed with a signature, so I asked him what it meant. He told me that this is a new movement to recognize the rights of transgender people who may biologically belong to one sex but psychologically identify as the other.

In other words, you could have been born with male genital organs but want to be called a woman or the other way around. I thanked him for informing me and totally respected this idea. I said to myself that I'm not one to judge anybody's right to self-determination and I will respect a person's wishes who wants to be called by a certain pronoun.

In later months, I saw a movement against this movement from those people who were opposed to transgenderism in any shape or form. Like so many other controversial issues in life, both sides have strong opinions and people with extreme views keep clashing with each other.

A couple of weeks ago, I was in a park enjoying an unseasonably pleasant evening. I had found a nice spot on the grass and was sitting there soaking up the sun and reading an engaging book. I was having a refreshing iced tea that I kept to my side between sips.

An elderly lady passed by, and she had the cutest puppy that was hopping around and was becoming the object of attention of anybody that was around in the park at that time. The puppy jumped close to me and started licking at the straw of my iced tea. The lady quickly jumped forward and apologized to me and pulled on the puppy's leash.

I wanted to say, "Don't worry, that's OK. It must be thirsty."

Although I had thought of these words to say in my mind, I hesitated because I could not bring myself to address the puppy by the pronoun "it." The puppy was like the lady's child and how would one feel if rather than asking if it's a boy or a girl, you call someone's child "it?"

At that moment, I tried to make the best estimate of what the gender of the puppy might be. It appeared nice and pretty. The colors were brown and black. The nose was cute, and the face was adorable but for the life of me, I could not guess the gender of the puppy. It could have been a male or a female. The genitals were not easily visible as it was happily hopping around.

I had to assign a gender and say something so I just went with my instinct and said, "It's OK, she must be thirsty."

"Sorry about that. He is just being impatient here. He is really enjoying the weather and has been running around a lot and that's why he is trying to drink anything that is coming his way!" was the dog owner's response.

They both left but I was left with an uneasy feeling that I used the wrong pronoun for the puppy. What if the lady did not like that, I used the wrong pronoun for the puppy? She must be thinking that I made an assumption based on the puppy's appearance which I should not have.

Maybe I should have used "it" for the puppy but that would have been even worse. After all, he was a puppy and not a lifeless toy. What if the puppy understood what was going on and got offended? Does it really matter?

We all know that dogs have feelings. They cry, and they frown. They feel pain; you can see it in their eyes. They get upset and angry. They smile and get excited when they see their owner-parent at the end of a long day when they come home from work.

Do dogs also feel embarrassed or offended if they are addressed with the "wrong" pronoun? If we care about all the rest of their feelings and emotions, should we also care about trying to know what their pronouns are?

When it comes to humans, if you ask a transgender person's parents, many of them will tell you that their children behaved in a transgender manner even before they developed a conscious thought process. Dog parents could perhaps say the same about the puppies and they would have an idea of the gender their dog-child identifies as.

In a world where human transgenderism still faces profound hostility, would it be all so crazy if the next time I meet a dog in a park or at the vet's office, and ask the owner, "What are your dog's pronouns?"

A Moment of Shame for a Pakistani Doctor

"A good doctor has to wear three hats. That of a clinician, a researcher, and that of a teacher." I remember being instructed by the Program Director on the first day of my residency training.

I always enjoyed the teaching aspect of medicine and am fortunate to work at an institution where I have the opportunity to teach students of all levels.

These range from trainees early in their careers such as medical and nursing students, residents, physician assistants, and nurse practitioners all the way up to fellows undergoing high-level specialty training.

While teaching, to make any topic interesting, one tip is to dig into the history of what is being taught. The history of medicine is a subject on its own and it is simply fascinating to learn how doctors used to treat patients since the beginning of time.

It is interesting to read about the then-prevailing theories and understanding, or the lack thereof, of human physiological and pathological mechanisms and how many advancements have been made in the last couple of centuries.

Antibiotics and vaccines that are responsible for saving millions of lives on a daily basis are relatively recent discoveries for mankind. The discovery that the heart is a pump responsible for the circulation of blood was made only a few hundred years ago.

The prevailing theory for centuries was that the human body is made up of four liquids (called humors in Latin); green, red, yellow, and black, and bodily functions are dependent on their harmonious balance. These are just a few examples of how fascinating the history of medicine is.

During rounds, it is not uncommon for me to look up online the stories behind certain clinical syndromes, where their names are derived from and other interesting historical pieces of information about the topic under discussion.

This particular morning, I was teaching the residents that there is only one device that has ever been invented in the history of medicine that is used to deliver chemotherapy into the area called the intrathecal or intraventricular space that carries the cerebrospinal fluid surrounding the brain and the spinal cord.

This is to either treat or prevent the spread of cancer into this area where drugs injected into the veins cannot enter because of the so-called "blood-brain barrier." The name of this device, which is used all around the world, is "Ommaya Reservoir."

Flanked by about half a dozen students, I turned around and pulled up the computer screen and typed in "history of Ommaya Reservoir" in the search bar. To my unexpected surprise, I came to find out that the device was named after its inventor Dr. Ayub Khan Ommaya. This name sounded like a very familiar Pakistani name to me.

When I read more about him, I came to find out that he was actually a Pakistani neurosurgeon who graduated from King Edward Medical College in Lahore and had an illustrious career at George Washington University in Washington, DC.

Suddenly, a feeling of profound shame hit me. Here I was, a Pakistani American medical oncologist having gone through medical school in Pakistan followed by years of training in medicine and then oncology at various institutions in the United States. I had used the Ommaya Reservoir countless times not knowing the origin of the device.

I was finding out by a random internet search that this device, a widely used instrument across the globe, was invented by a doctor who had walked in the same footsteps as I did.

I felt betrayed by my Pakistani medical education system for not highlighting this piece of information in our curriculum.

I read more about him. Born in Mian Channu, Punjab in 1930 to a Pakistani Muslim father and a French Catholic mother, Dr. Ayub Khan Ommaya became a Rhodes Scholar and was accepted to study at the Oxford University.

He later progressed on to work at the prestigious National Institute of Health in Bethesda, Maryland and became a professor of Neurosurgery at the George Washington University.

Not only did he invent the Ommaya Reservoir, but he was also an expert in the field of traumatic brain injuries and his work had special importance in the establishment of the National Center for Injury Prevention and Control at the Centers for Disease Control (CDC.)

He was an interesting character in that he was also an opera singer and used to sing for his patients after finishing surgeries, earning him the nickname of the "singing neurosurgeon."

In his younger years, he won the National Swimming Championship in Pakistan and was also in the rowing team at Balliol College in Oxford. In his later years, he developed Alzheimer's disease and moved back to Pakistan. He eventually died in Islamabad.

If you look at the history of medicine, for the last couple of centuries, most of the diseases and syndromes were named after either the doctor who discovered them for the first time or occasionally named after the patients. Surgical operations were also routinely named after pioneering surgeons.

These eponymous practices have now been mostly discontinued in the favor of giving more technically accurate names to newly discovered diseases and procedures. In today's world, it has become quite unique to have a medical device named after a person.

There are a number of such devices and catheters that are used to gain access to the arteries and veins and other organs of the body but to date, the Ommaya Reservoir remains to be the only device that can be used to gain access to inject chemotherapy or antibiotics into the cerebrospinal fluid.

Having mixed emotions – of pride on one hand but the shame of ignorance on the other, I started asking around.

I went to multiple other Pakistani-origin doctors and asked them if they knew who Dr. Ayub Khan Ommaya was. All I encountered were blank faces and they were equally surprised as I was to find out about the origins of this device. I called up a couple of friends who were graduates of King Edwardes Medical College and asked them if they knew about Dr. Ommaya.

Since he was a graduate of the same medical school, I thought that they may have a higher chance of knowing about him but unfortunately, no one knew of him. I thought that maybe this was very specific to Oncology or Neurosurgery and other fields of medicine might not know much about him, but none of my colleagues from those specialties knew about him.

I still do not have an answer as to why Dr. Ayub Khan Ommaya is relatively obscure in the Pakistani medical community. In the current times, most of the cutting-edge research and new advancements in medicine are happening in the United States, followed by Europe.

In this climate, for a Pakistani doctor to invent a device that is used across the world and for it to be the only device used for this indication is a pretty big deal.

Why is his name not included in our medical curriculum? Why isn't there a chapter about him in our medical books? Why aren't there lecture halls or auditoriums named after him? Why aren't grants and scholarships named after him? Why is he an anonymous figure for the doctors of the whole country?

A quote attributed to Abraham Lincoln goes, "A nation that does not honor its heroes, will not long endure." The anonymity of Dr. Ommaya's name amongst the medical fraternity of Pakistan is nothing less than a matter of neglect and shame for us.

I hereby make a petition to the College of Physicians and Surgeons of Pakistan to include a mandatory chapter in the medical curriculum of Pakistan. How else do we expect to produce and present more Ommayas to the world?

We need more Black Cops, we need more Black Physicians

I am neither black nor white. I'm brown. I can choose to stay silent and indifferent, but the human and the American in me urges me to express my feelings and opinion about the current situation in the country resulting from a series of unfortunate events, particularly George Floyd's blatant murder in broad daylight.

I immigrated to this great country about fifteen years ago. From a distance, I had a very superficial idea of the race issues confronting America, but it was only after living here and witnessing events first-hand that I realized how deep-rooted the racial conflicts are.

When Barack Obama took his first oath as President, it was a proud moment for me as an immigrant father. I still remember telling my then five years old daughter, "you, my child, were born in this country, and you can one day become the President of the United States."

Little did I know that only a few years later, she would come crying to me because someone at school told her that Donald Trump was not letting any Muslims in the country and that she thought that she would have to leave America.

You might say that religious discrimination is different than racism, but you get the point. I tried to console her and tell her right from wrong, but I felt helpless because her mind was too immature to understand the depth of arguments.

As a physician, I had the chance to rotate through different clinics catering to different classes of society. These ranged from upscale clinics in the suburbs where the patients were highly privileged, flying in from different states, staying at nearby luxury hotels to obtain second and third opinions. Then there were inner-city clinics providing care to the indigent and uninsured.

I was proud to feel that the medical care and recommendations that both the groups received from us were exactly similar, and our decisions and service for them were the same regardless of their ethnicity or socioeconomic status.

But I was still able to notice some areas in medicine where the care was not equal for different ethnic groups. During my hematology training (fellowship), I came to know that it is important for the donor cells to be as close of a match to the recipient not only for a successful transplant but also to prevent graft-versus-host disease.

It was also intriguing that the ethnicity mattered since there was more of a chance for a better match if both donor and recipient were of the same race.

It was shocking to find out that if you are a white patient, the chances of finding a white donor are 8 out of 10, but if you are a black patient, the chances of finding a black donor are only 2 out of 10!

I felt that I wanted to do something about this statistic. I contacted the National Bone Marrow Donation Registry and obtained information and materials to organize bone marrow donation drives. However, my goal was to target only the minorities, specifically the black community.

Through patients and friends, I was able to arrange these drives in black churches and at black community events. I created an easy-to-understand power-point presentation explaining the complex transplant process.

I hoped that if I, as a man of color myself, instead of a white physician, stood in front of them, they would relate and volunteer to become stem cell donors, but I could still see their eyes filled with suspicion.

Perhaps they were wondering how the cheek swabs would be exploited by the medical community reminiscent of Henrietta Lacks' cervical cancer cells or the images of the patients undergoing the Tuskegee atrocity flashed in their minds. Maybe the thoughts of the brutal procedures conducted by James Sims came back to haunt them.

I still feel that we have come a long way to remedy the racial discrimination in medicine, but we still have not been able to win the trust of the black community.

Research practices have been significantly improvised and well-monitored to ensure that ethnic injustice is not done, but we would also be very naïve to think that we can erase the memory of those events that easily.

Another disease that brings to light the racial disparity in medicine is the sickle cell disease. This disease is more common in the black population. It is a devastating disease to have, and life can be miserable with repeated episodes of painful crises that are often misunderstood as narcotic drug-seeking behavior.

Nowhere else is medicine can you find an example of the treatment of a disease resulting in another more serious condition, in this case, treatment with narcotics leading to iatrogenic opioid addiction.

When it comes to medical research, there is a significant lack of medical research for this disease, and for decades, no significant breakthroughs have taken place except for a couple of oral medications (such as hydroxyurea) showing benefit.

There is a lack of comprehensive clinics for patients with sickle cell disease. I am a practicing hematologist, and I often find it incredibly difficult to do justice to the care of sickle cell patients due to lack of resources.

No mention of atrocities against black people can be justified without a word of support for the majority of white cops who get a bad name and are placed in harm's way only because of the discrimination exhibited by a few. 9/11 was perpetrated by a handful of so-called Muslims in the name of Islam, but only the ignorant held billions of Muslims around the world responsible.

How can we, as physicians, gain the trust of our black patients? It will take time.

I feel that we are doing a lot of right things by delivering care and compassion without discrimination, but one thing that will have a profound impact is if we have a much higher number of black physicians and medical researchers.

It will be much easier for a black patient to trust a black doctor, and this way, trust will build in the profession in general. Black population will be better represented in research studies.

Perhaps there should be significant cuts in student fees for medical school for black students, and further incentives and allowances should be made.

We need more black cops. We need more black physicians.

Some Gifts From a Dying Man

Born with a Bad Liver

I am fortunate in that there are about a dozen of us who have been buddies since we were in kindergarten. When we were growing up, they would keep the kids in the same class across the years.

That way, in every class, a group of friends had gone to the same classroom for up to twelve years in a row, from kindergarten until they graduated high school.

This group became another family on top of the family you had in the first place, and in many ways, occupied your mind and activities more than your biological family.

Not everybody I have met can tell me they have a close group of friends like that. Or a group of friends that they have been friends with for more than just a few years.

When my kids went to school, I was quite surprised to find out that they shuffle the kids each year so that no kids remain in the same classroom throughout their time in school.

The proponents of this arrangement claim that the kids become more adaptable to change and end up making a wider group of friends. But there is no denying the fact that the close bond one would make with a group that you shared the classroom with all these years is not possible to make when you keep changing classmates.

One of my friends from my earliest days of life is Asad. At that time, he was the kind of kid who stood out so much for being adorable that his becoming an instant center of attraction amongst a group of kids was not unusual. But there was a problem.

When he was born, the right side of his abdomen protruded outwards as if some organ was trying to push out of his body. The doctors told his parents that he had an enlarged liver. He used to turn yellow as a banana every few weeks, and the doctors had to give him medicine to treat the jaundice.

His parents took him to several different pediatricians, but they were having difficulty making an accurate diagnosis. Since his episodes of jaundice would improve after a few days of medications and did not limit his growth, his parents, in a way, got used to it and thought that he would grow out of it like other diseases that some children grow out of.

They were wrong, unfortunately. When he was in high school, he had another attack of jaundice, and this was accompanied by severe pain in the right side of the abdomen.

They took him to the emergency room, and the doctors did some tests urgently and explained to them that he had developed swelling and infection of his gall bladder and he had to undergo emergent surgery.

The surgeon happened to be the father of another friend of ours, and Asad's parents were reassured that he was in good hands. Before taking him to the operating room, he told them to expect the operation to be not more than a couple of hours, but it took them close to ten hours to finish the operation.

The surgeon later explained that when they opened his abdomen, they saw a large cyst that was pushing upon multiple organs and, in doing so, causing obstruction in the bile ducts. He was able to remove the large cyst and, along with it, had to remove part of the intestine, too.

Already exhausted from all the worrying and the praying while their son was being operated upon for so many hours, they sighed with relief that the operation was successful and hoped that this should be the end of his jaundice attacks that he had been going through since being born.

For a few months, he had to stay home to recover from the long operation. One morning, he woke up jaundiced yet again.

They took him back to the doctors who had given up on any further diagnostic studies by then. A physician who had trained in England suggested that he be taken to London, where a hepatobiliary specialist could see him.

Asad's father was not poor, but he wasn't extraordinarily wealthy either. He had a good position in a reputable bank, but other than his salary, he did not have other means, such as inherited assets, to rely on.

But it was becoming a matter of life or death for his son. Somehow, he managed to gather enough money from his savings and some help from close friends and family, and they took him to London.

The doctors in London did additional tests and suggested that he probably had a stricture or a cyst in his bile ducts and offered another operation.

He underwent this operation without difficulty and returned home only to find out a few weeks later that the bouts of jaundice kept recurring. Feelings of hopelessness began to take root since nobody seemed to know the solution to the problem.

Doctors suggested that he undergo a liver transplant, but this service was not available in Pakistan. They inquired about the costs in the United States and the United Kingdom only to find out that this was not even fathomable. The costs in China were relatively low but still far beyond the reach of a middle-class family from Pakistan.

The episodes of jaundice had now started becoming more complicated. Asad was now in his twenties. He started getting severe pain that would start from his upper abdomen and move to his upper back. He started to take pain medicine more frequently.

Sometimes, the pain would be so severe that he had to go to the emergency room to receive intravenous pain medications. The frequency of the episodes intensified. This now became complicated by the swelling in his legs and in his abdomen.

He was put on diuretics, and his shoes did not fit him anymore. He gained a lot of weight, which was all fluid weight, and his abdomen got swollen to the point that his usual clothes did not fit him anymore.

One day, as he was going through a similar painful episode when he was taken to the emergency room, he lost consciousness. The doctors did some tests and let the family know that his liver had now completely failed.

They admitted him to the intensive care unit and started multiple infusions. After a few hours, the doctors started having end-of-life discussions and asked them to call any family members who were close to him to say their goodbyes.

While this was happening, Asad's parents were told about a new doctor who had recently arrived to establish his practice after finishing his training in the United Kingdom. They made a frantic phone call to him, and he suggested the name of a doctor from India who was highly reputed as a successful liver transplant surgeon.

He suggested that, as a last-ditch effort, Asad be taken to Chennai, India, to see if his life could be saved.

They quickly acquired all the information and got in touch with the hospital in Chennai. They were very good about guiding them through the whole process. They would search Asad's family for a suitable donor and then take a part of the family member's liver and transplant it into Asad. Asad's father was not found to be a suitable donor because he had fatty liver.

However, Asad's brother, who was only a few years younger, was found to be a suitable donor. As much as Asad's parents were hopeful, they had to go through the mental agony of the prospect of having not only one but two of their sons undergo major surgeries at the same time.

The cost that would be associated with the liver transplant in India was still very high. Asad's father sold his car, and his mother sold all her jewelry. His officemates started a funding drive, and they generated enough funds to be able to afford the transplant. They rushed to the embassy and got visas to travel to India.

When all the arrangements were made, Asad was transported straight from the hospital to the airport. He arrived in Chennai and was admitted to the hospital. They took 60% of his brother's liver and transplanted it into Asad.

Asad spent four months hospitalized in India but started showing signs of recovery. His pain improved, and his swelling went away. They kept worrying that any day, he would wake up with another bout of jaundice, but fortunately, the attacks disappeared.

He recovered to the point of being able to travel back home. He was started on medications to suppress his immune system so that his brother's liver would not be rejected by his body.

Asad has been living without any complications of the transplant so far. He is happily married and has three beautiful children. He has a good job, enjoys life like any of us, and does not have to worry about getting sick every few months. A liver transplant from his brother brought him back to normal life from a state when the doctors had given up on him.

Skip the Question

When I was growing up in Pakistan, organ donation was not something that I knew existed. No medical facilities would be competent enough to perform organ harvesting and donation.

Yes, blood transfusions were very common, but there was a lack of blood banking facilities, so it was not uncommon for people to have to find compatible blood on their own. This was done by mass text messages and word of mouth.

It was also a common sight at busy intersections to see people holding placards asking for a specific type of blood group. Other than Asad's story, I do not have any other transplant story among the people that I know.

The first time I gave a thought to organ donation was when I immigrated to America. After passing the driving test in a rental car in Dallas, Texas, I sat down to fill out the final form to obtain my license.

At the end of the form, there was a line with a lengthy question asking whether I wanted to be added to the organ donation registry. Instead of the Yes and No options, the options were Yes and Skip This Question.

I was in a hurry and wanted to quickly fill out the form so that I could submit it and go on with the rest of my day. I checked off Skip This Question and submitted the form.

I could have forgotten about it because you can't live your life chasing every dumb question on any form that you fill. But on the other hand, I am also not the type of person who likes to skip questions. I will tell you if I know the answer or not. I wouldn't keep you hanging by skipping a question.

I kept thinking about it. I had never thought about whether I wanted to donate my organs or not. I thought about how it would work.

When I die, they will have a team of doctors cut me all open and take out my lungs, kidneys, liver, heart, and eyes, and then sew me back up. I would be dead, so I wouldn't feel anything. Or would I?

What if it is my perception that after death, my body would not feel anything, but what if my perception is wrong? As a human, how can I be so sure of anything? How can anybody be so sure?

What if my family does not want me to go through such a procedure? What if they go through such emotional trauma by knowing what the doctors are doing to my body? They may not be able to bear it.

But I would be doing such a noble deed. I would literally be saving lives.

Two people will not need dialysis. Two people who cannot breathe on their own would be able to breathe because of me. One person with a failed heart will live on, thanks to my heart. Two blind people will see again.

That is more good than I have ever done in my life. How can I not sign up for organ donation? I will be gone, but my organs will live on for another many years. The prayers of the recipients and their families would ensure a pretty successful afterlife.

Still, before committing to become an organ donor, I asked around. I found out that people were quite divided on this issue.

As many people as I found out had signed up to be donors, I also found many people who had decided not to become organ donors. Some people also told me that they were not sure if their religion allowed organ donation. I looked up several religions and found that most religions around the world currently allow organ donation.

So I figured that if someone is deciding not to donate based on religious reasons, they probably either misunderstand their own religion's teachings or belong to quite a small school of thought within their religious rankings.

After a few years, when it was time to renew my driver's license, I checked Yes on the organ donation question on the form. I felt good about it.

I hoped that I would never be in a situation where that had to happen, but if it happened, my organs would be put to good use, and I would be very happy about it in some way.

Learning Hematology at the N.I.H.

Over the years, I finally entered the field of Hematology, the medical specialty that makes you an expert at blood. There are several important organs in the body, and the specialty of every organ is very interesting.

But blood traverses every nook and corner of your body, so to be a good hematologist, you have to have a very good understanding of all the organs through which blood runs.

As part of hematology training, we spent a month in the bone marrow transplant department. The hospital where I was training in Washington D.C. had contracted with the National Institute of Health (NIH), so the hematology fellows got to spend about a month of training time on the transplant floor at the NIH.

For those not familiar with the NIH, it is the largest government-run medical research institute in the entire world. It was located a few miles away in Bethesda, Maryland.

Call it my naivety, but when my rotation was about to start, instead of being excited, I was more worried about how I would get there. D.C. traffic was already a nightmare. Whether you drive or take public transportation like the tube or the bus, it is equally difficult and time-consuming.

On my first day, as I drove into the NIH, I found myself in a sprawling complex of buildings trying to look for the administration office from where I had to get my ID badge.

By this time, I had already worked in several different hospitals across the Northeast of the USA, but this was the first time I was entering a campus that covered 300 acres.

By the time I reached the bone marrow transplant building, I was already late for rounds, making a horrible first impression. The team that I was going to work with was very nice, though, and made me feel comfortable right away. They showed me around, explained the daily routine, and made me familiar with their electronic health record system.

There was a lot to learn from that rotation. Working at the NIH was also a once-in-a-lifetime kind of experience. I still did not fully realize the significance of working there until after my fellowship was over.

It hit me specifically when, several years later in 2020, during the peak of the COVID pandemic, Dr. Anthony Fauci resurfaced in the international limelight as the infectious disease expert leading the fight against the disease.

His personality was revered in the scientific community, but he became the target of hate and slander amongst the political and conspiracy theory-mongering community.

I read a short biography about him in the New Yorker and found out that he had to undergo similar treatment from the masses during the HIV epidemic days a few decades ago.

In the article, I read that he has worked out of the same office throughout his career at one of the infectious disease buildings on the NIH campus. This was only a few buildings away from the bone marrow transplant center where I had done my rotation.

Hailing from a third-world country where medical research was nearly non-existent, I was able to reach a point where I could get expert training in a complex medical field at such a highly prestigious institution, which gave me a sense of high achievement and honor.

During my time at the NIH, I got to work with highly intellectual people coming from all over the world. I worked with highly qualified hematologists, infectious disease specialists, and transplant doctors. The amount of knowledge and sense of inquiry that each individual possessed was unlike any other place that I have worked at.

Even an afternoon discussion over lunch with some of the Professors felt like attending in-depth lectures on whatever topic was under discussion.

The weekly grand rounds were at a scientific level that was often beyond my comprehension.

The scientists delivering those lectures were well-known across the world and lead authors of papers from Nature and Science. No wonder that, to date, research done at the NIH has garnered more than 150 Nobel prizes.

I learned a lot about bone marrow transplants during my time training at the NIH. Here, for the reader who is not a physician, allow me to explain some of the basics of a bone marrow transplant. The way I explain it to my patients is to first bring their attention to what bone marrow is. I give the following spiel routinely in my clinic:

"America is a big meat-eating nation, but the butchers throw away the fat and the bone marrow. That is why a lot of my patients say that they have never even seen bone marrow. Where I grew up, in the northern part of Pakistan, you pay extra to add bone marrow to your beef patties. In Mexico, I have often seen large shafts of bones cut longitudinally with bone marrow intact and cooked in it, served as a delicacy.

So, it is a spongy liquid substance present inside our bones. This is where our blood is made. If you have ever wondered where all the blood comes from in our body, the bone marrow is where it is made. If you take a drop of blood and look at it under the microscope, it is made of three different types of cells called red cells, white cells, and platelets, all of which have vital functions in our body and are all manufactured inside the bone marrow."

When bone marrow makes these blood cells, the first cell that is born is called a "stem" cell, which then differentiates into all these other kinds of blood cells. So to say, the stem cell is a parent cell that has the capacity to turn into any kind of blood cell.

When someone gets a disease of the bone marrow, such as leukemia, lymphoma, or myeloma, the bone marrow starts making abnormal cells. That is when, to cure that disease, the only option is to replace the bone marrow with somebody else's marrow. That is done through a process called a bone marrow transplant.

Although a bone marrow transplant can save someone's life by curing leukemia, the recipient's immune system can attack it since, of course, it belongs to another person and leads to a serious disease called Graft Versus Host disease, which in itself could be life-threatening or lead to a seriously impaired quality of life.

When doctors transplant any other organ from one person to another, such as a liver or a kidney, it involves performing an operation and taking that organ out of the donor and surgically transplanting it into the recipient. Since bone marrow cells are in liquid form, such an operation is not performed.

The bone marrow cells are obtained from the donor by sticking a needle in the hip bone and aspirating a large number of bone marrow cells into a bag that looks exactly like a bag of blood.

This is then infused into the recipient via intravenous administration, and the cells find their way to the bone marrow, settle down, and start growing, a process called engraftment.

As I saw patients upon patients with serious blood disorders getting bone marrow transplants, I realized that none of these patients would have any hope of staying alive or being cured unless another person somewhere had not decided to become a bone marrow donor.

There was a time when the stem cell registry process was not as established as it is today, so the only hope was to turn to family members for donation.

A patient's friends and family had to either volunteer themselves or run a local bone marrow donation drive to find someone who would be willing to donate. You could still find someone as a donor, albeit with a lot of difficulty, but the stem cell type had to be very similar.

There are certain markers on these cells called the HLA markers, and if these are not a good match to the recipient, then there would be significant problems with the success of the transplant, which would also lead to serious symptoms from Graft versus Host disease.

Here, I also stumbled upon a startling fact involving the donor's race and ethnicity versus the recipient. Come to find out that for other organs such as a kidney or the liver etc., the race of the donor does not matter, but when it comes to bone marrow cells, there is more of a chance of being a perfect HLA match if the race of the donor and the recipient is similar.

In today's America, if you are a White/Caucasian person, the chances that you can get a perfect match are as high as about 9 out of 10.

But if you are Black, you only have 2 to 3 out of 10 chances to find a perfect match. The percentages of other ethnicities finding a good match are somewhere in the middle of those numbers.

Signing up as a bone marrow donor

By this time, I was almost ready to sign up as a bone marrow donor. I went to the "Be The Match" website, which had all the information about the donation process.

The process would involve signing up at the website, and they would send you a kit. The kit would have a swab that looked exactly like a Q-tip, which you were supposed to rub inside your cheek, label it, and send it back. That seemed easy enough.

They would analyze your cells, obtain your HLA information, and store it in the registry that contained similar samples from hundreds of thousands of other potential donors.

At any time, anywhere in the country, if anybody developed leukemia or other such diseases that required a bone marrow transplant, they would run their samples against the registry, and whoever was found to be the best or 10 out of 10 match, would be selected.

If multiple samples were found to be the best match, then they would contact the donors and obtain their medical history. They would typically choose younger and healthier donors since their cells would be considered more suitable for a successful transplant.

As a donor, if you were found to be the perfect match, the registry would contact you, and they would ask if you were still in a situation to donate.

If you agreed, then you would have to take a few days off of work; that would most likely be an unpaid leave, or you would have to take it from your own vacation time. You would go to a local hospital, and the doctors would obtain your bone marrow cells and send them to the recipient.

This is where I had to pause while reading about the procedure. I would have loved to sign up as a donor and save somebody's life someday, but what would I do about the fact that I absolutely hate needles?

So much is my aversion to needles that I often find myself finding excuses to postpone my dental appointments. My dentist probably hates me but doesn't say it to my face.

When he has to drill holes in my teeth, even before his tools touch my mouth, my whole body tenses up, and I start clenching my jaw, and I start involuntarily withdrawing my body away from him.

He repeatedly asks me to relax, and I tell him to try to ignore me and keep doing his job. Every time I have to have dental work done, it's a struggle for both him and me.

With such a phobia of needles and pain, how would I even be able to become a bone marrow donor? I started looking more into the process of how I would donate if called.

The traditional way of obtaining stem cells from the donor is by drilling a large bone marrow biopsy needle (called the Jamshidi needle) into the hip bone and sucking (aspirating) bone marrow directly from there. This sounded to me like a torture method from the medieval times.

During hematology training, everybody has to learn how to aspirate bone marrow. You literally take this long and wide needle, have the patient lie down on their stomach, identify their hip bone, and puncture their skin after applying some local anesthesia.

Then, with the tip of the needle, you find the hard bone surface and start pushing and drilling the needle right into it. The patient starts moaning, and it is not uncommon for some patients to start screaming.

The worst is when your needle is all the way inside the marrow, and you pull on the syringe to aspirate it. The doctor even says at this time, "This will be the worst part."

After the procedure is done, you apply the band-aid after the bleeding stops, and typically, there isn't much residual pain after the procedure, but the memory of the pain lingers to scar the patient for the rest of his life.

I asked one of my hematology attendings if they knew how they obtained bone marrow cells for a transplant.

"Well, you know how you do a bone marrow biopsy? It is done very similarly except for the fact that in a simple bone marrow biopsy, you just go into one side of the hip bone, stick the needle once, and aspirate a small sample of bone marrow - just enough to analyze the sample and come to a diagnosis. In a donation process, typically, two doctors will stand on either side of the donor and stick in the bone marrow needles multiple times and keep aspirating until they have enough stem cells that would be required for a successful transplant," he replied.

I became quite squeamish just by listening to the procedure and I responded that there was no way that I could go through that.

He looked at me reassuringly and told me they would most likely do it under general anesthesia. I wasn't sold.

"Well, if you are that worried, then you can ask for your bone marrow cells to be taken by the apheresis method," he suggested.

"How does that work?" I inquired.

"They give you these injections in the belly for a few days, and the way they work is that your stem cells are released from the bone marrow into the blood in your veins. After a few days of injections, they will put an IV in your arm and hook you up to a machine called an apheresis machine and obtain your blood. They have the capacity to filter your blood and take the needed amount of stem cells and give your blood back to you," he explained.

"This seems like a much more doable procedure compared to the medieval torture method you were explaining earlier," I said with some relief.

"There can still be some pain because as those stem cells are released from the bone marrow, sometimes the bones can become very achy to the point that you may have to take some pain medicine," he warned.

"I think it still sounds better than the alternative," I said.

By now, I had finalized my decision to sign up as a bone marrow donor.

"You crazy. Don't do it!"

I was amazed at how long it took me to commit myself to becoming a donor. I entered all my information in the "Be The Match" registry website, and a few days later, as I was going to work, I opened my mailbox, and there it was, a package with their insignia on it.

I did not yet open it as I was getting late to work and had to struggle in traffic for almost an hour. That was my commute to work while living in Washington, D.C.

As I arrived at work, I settled down in front of a work computer and quickly reviewed the overnight information about all my patients that I had to present during morning rounds. I still had about ten minutes before the rounds would start, so I pulled out the package from my bag, put it on the table in front of me, and began to open it.

As the contents spilled out of the package, I saw that there were a number of pamphlets with all the information about the whole process of bone marrow donation. There was also a return envelope that said, 'No stamp necessary if mailed within the United States.'

Then came out a test tube along with an instructional card and a couple of swabs that looked like q tips. I read the instructions. I had to take a swab and rub it inside my cheek for a few seconds to make sure that adequate cells transferred onto it, and then I had to put it back in the tube, close it, seal it in the envelope, and put it back in the mail.

As I brought the swab closer to my mouth, I heard someone say my name. "Farhan! What are you doing?"

It was Ming. He was another Hematology fellow from China who was also doing his training at the NIH. Based on our schedules, we spent the month together at the bone marrow transplant unit at the NIH.

Unlike myself, where it was my first encounter working at a bone marrow unit, he had already done a PhD in hematology and molecular biology in China.

He was already an experienced and accomplished hematologist in his own country and was selected out of a huge number of applicants for a fully paid scholarship to come get some additional training at the NIH.

He was collaborating with the faculty at the NIH on several projects and, a few days earlier, had told me how he would get at least a dozen publications in highly sought-after peer-reviewed medical journals both in the United States and in China.

During medical rounds, the NIH attendings would often ask for his opinion in his areas of expertise, making him feel like a colleague rather than a student.

He would often explain difficult cases to me, and I would, in return, help him navigate the electronic health record and tell him which bars to go to on the weekend.

The cheek swab was in midair, and I was bringing it close to my mouth when I paused and looked back at him.

"I'm signing up as a bone marrow donor," I explained to him what I was doing.

"You crazy. Don't do it!" He warned me.

I was very surprised at what he said, and my mind quickly thought of a few reasons why he was stopping me from doing it.

Was it because the rounds were about to start, and I would not be able to collect a sample properly in a rush?

Was it because he was suggesting that I donate in a different way such as via a bone marrow biopsy harvest or was it because there might be some other way for me to send the sample such as in-person rather than by mail?

"Why? What happened?" I asked.

"They give you growth factor to collect your stem cells. You get leukemia from growth factor. You become doctor and help so many people get transplant. But if you get leukemia, then you can't help all these patients," he explained.

I literally froze right there in my shoes.

Never had I imagined that this was a concern. I thought that I had already researched this topic and had read everything about it that I could find online and in any print materials.

Nowhere was it even mentioned as a myth or any kind of concern that growth factor could cause leukemia. But if Ming was saying it, there must be some truth to it, and I had to look further into it.

"But I never heard of it. Is it true? How do you know this?" I asked.

"Yes, there are some reports of it. Studies have not proven it, but they have not disproven it either," he said.

The cheek swab was halfway in the air from the package to my mouth as we were having this conversation. I found myself bringing it slowly back to the packet, without swabbing my cheek and put the packet back in my work bag.

As soon as I had a chance, I went back online and started browsing about any link between growth factor and leukemia.

I found small studies suggesting the link but did not find any major clinical trials establishing a clear link between the two.

I thought to myself that if it were such a definite risk, so many people would not sign up as bone marrow donors, and the doctors would discourage people from becoming donors, but that was clearly not the case.

I also thought that although Ming was a highly accomplished academic and was already an expert in this field, there must be some truth to what he was saying, but what if it was just a mythical belief that he had bought into and I should forget about what he was saying and stick to my initial intention of becoming a donor and save somebody's life.

But every time I went back to making my decision to send my cheek swab to the registry, his words would echo in my mind, "You crazy, you get growth factor, you get leukemia."

It bothered me for several years that I had gotten so close to becoming a donor, but I had changed my intention at the last moment. I discussed this with several of my other hematology colleagues, who all assured me that becoming a donor was the right thing to do.

I thought that the chances of me getting leukemia from the growth factor would be minuscule, but on the other hand, the opportunity to save somebody's life would bring such fulfillment and a sense of beneficence that I eventually was able to make my final decision.

I opted to have another kit delivered to me and sent my cheek swabs, and I am now a part of the registry.

After I finished my training, I started working as a hematologist at a job that I loved. I was well-settled and had a good work-life balance. I had a high level of professional satisfaction, but I was looking for volunteer work.

"You should be ashamed of yourself for doing this to our children."

Although I was grateful that medicine is a profession in which you end up helping people on your job, I wanted to do something for people for which I did not get paid. I asked around and researched online what kinds of volunteer work I could do.

This is when one fact that I had learned during my training kept repeating in my mind.

The fact that if you are Black in America, you only have about two out of ten chances of matching with a perfect donor if you need a bone marrow transplant. Something inside me wanted to do something to help with that statistic.

I decided to contact the NMDP (National Marrow Donor Program) bone marrow registry and ask them if I could arrange and run bone marrow donation drives in the community.

My thought was that I would go to only Black or other ethnic minority groups and spread awareness about the process, and even if I was able to convince a handful of people to sign up as donors, I would have played my part.

The NMDP representative was very encouraging, and he sent me a big box of materials to help arrange such a donation drive. This included pamphlets, brochures, and other materials with all the information printed on them.

I contacted a patient of mine who had gone through a successful bone marrow transplant herself and who was very socially active in her community.

I told her about my intentions, and she was very helpful in setting up a time for me at her church. I prepared a short presentation and gave information to all the attendees.

At the end of the presentation, a couple of people also came up to the desk that I had set up and signed up as donors. I felt accomplished and encouraged but realized that it was not an easy task.

It did require taking out time from your personal time, setting up an information desk, and trying to do a lot of teaching and convincing, but then this is what a donation drive was all about.

After speaking at a few black churches, I ran out of contacts to find out where to go and hold any future bone marrow donation drives. I once also got a stall at the local African American Convention in downtown, and this also generated a few donor signups.

My kids were little at that time, in elementary school, and I would take them with me. For them, it was an enjoyable experience because they felt like they were doing something very important.

I thought that other than the black community, I could also go to gathering places of other ethnic minorities and spread awareness. I came across Ahmat, a friend and colleague of mine who was a Turkish Cardiologist.

He appeared to be quite active in his community and once had asked me for a donation for the new Turkish mosque that his community was building in town. I called him up and asked him if I could run a bone marrow donation drive at his mosque. Eid was coming in a few weeks, and I knew that the attendance at the event would be pretty good.

He was more than helpful and told me that I could come to the mosque and set up a table, and he would even have it announced in Turkish during the sermon before the prayer.

I dressed up in Eid clothes and gathered my materials for the donation drive. I arrived early at the mosque. They provided me with a table and some chairs that were placed in the courtyard. It was a beautiful summer morning.

I set up the information materials on the table and neatly attached several signup sheets to the clipboards. Ahmat greeted me warmly and asked me if I needed anything else.

"Man, look at you! Is this how you are going to spend your Eid day?" He was implying that I was performing a very noble deed by dedicating my holiday to running a donation drive.

"Well, this is in the spirit of Eid. We should all do something like this from time to time to give back to the community," I replied.

As people started arriving, before they entered the mosque, they would look toward my table to figure out what I was there for. Some people would stop, and I would try to hand them pamphlets containing information about the bone marrow transplant process and how to become donors.

For most people, it was something beyond their comprehension, and they had puzzled looks on their faces. On top of that, there was a language barrier, and I realized that I should have tried to have some of that information translated into the Turkish language. Nonetheless, I kept doing my best to spread as much information as I could.

In about an hour's time, although dozens of people had stopped at my desk, only a couple of them had signed up. I wasn't particularly looking at the numbers, and although it would have been nice if a lot of people had signed up, it was not like I was selling something.

I thought that even if I spread awareness, people may understand the process and may be better prepared to sign up as donors in the future.

Meanwhile, Ahmat was walking around and attending to different tasks at the mosque. He was one of the managers and made sure that the seating and parking arrangements were running smoothly.

He passed by my desk and asked me if I needed anything. He saw people passing by and not stopping at my desk and felt that he needed to help me.

He went inside the mosque and rounded up a few young boys who appeared to be in their late teens and early twenties and asked them to come to my desk and sign up as donors.

I welcomed the young boys to my table and started handing over the informational pamphlets. As I was sitting there, a Turkish couple in their fifties passed us by. The husband was dressed up in charming, impeccably ironed clothes, and the wife was wearing a beautiful headscarf.

Unlike other people who did not have much of an idea about what was going on, this couple actually stopped and looked at the NBMD logo displayed on my table. They were saying something to each other while repeatedly looking back at me. Looking at their faces, it appeared that they were concerned or upset about something.

"Hello, here is some information about how to become bone marrow donors. Please let me know if you have any questions," I handed over a pamphlet to them.

"We know what this is all about, and you should be ashamed of yourself for doing this to our children. We will talk to the managers of the mosque who let you do this here on Eid day." The Turkish woman in the head scarf exclaimed.

This was a moment of extreme confusion for me.

Here I was, spending my free time trying to help a noble cause and there was this woman who was scolding me. Either she misunderstood what I was doing or there was some other aspect of this process that I was not comprehending.

With a very puzzled look on my face, I asked, "What do you mean? I am just running a bone marrow donation drive."

"We know exactly what you are doing, and this has brought a lot of conflict in our family," she replied.

I asked them to sit down and tell me more about what had happened.

"We moved to America eight years ago. Our son had barely turned eighteen years of age. We were in a new country, learning the language and other ways of life. We had a very happy life in Turkey and never even wanted to come here, but due to some conflict in our country, we had to leave because our lives were endangered. In that sense, we are thankful to this country for taking us in as refugees, but our hearts never left our country," she began telling her story.

"After we moved, we all struggled because of the new ways of life and the new language. But at least we were in safe housing and receiving enough benefits so that our children did not go to bed hungry at night. The kids were enrolled in a local school and were assimilated into the new society much faster and easier than us. We were still waiting for some members of our family to join us here because we knew that their lives were in danger in our homeland."

"One day, my son came back home, and he had similar pamphlets in his school bag. I asked him about it, and he told me that he had signed up as a bone marrow donor. We had no idea what he was talking about. He said that someone like you had come to the school, and most of the kids did not understand what this was all about, but the teachers were saying that this was to save someone's life.

Several of his friends put their names and phone numbers on the list, and my son did not want to feel left out, so he also signed up. We were worried about what he might have entered his name into, but since we also did not understand, we just let it pass. We thought of contacting the school, but life got busy, and we forgot all about it."

She was telling me her story while her husband was standing right behind her with a serious look on his face but not uttering a single word himself.

"A few months later, my son got a call from an American woman who said that she was calling from the same agency whose logo is on your poster, NMDP (National Marrow Donor Program.) She told him that there was someone in California who had leukemia, and our son's cells had been found to be the best match for the patient. They wanted to bring him into the hospital and keep going for a week to receive some sort of injections in his belly, and then they would hook him up to this big machine and take his blood."

My son initially did not tell us and took a couple of weeks to try to decide. He would have to skip school, and they told him that he would have pain in his bones when he received the injection and may even need to take pain medications. He knew that if he told us, we would never allow him to do something like that, but he could not go through the whole process without us knowing. We would have to find out.

The woman kept on calling him and telling him that the leukemia patient in California was waiting and that his life was dependent on him since they could not find any other suitable donor for him. Finally, he told us, and we were so mad.

How could they make little kids with immature minds do something like this? If a kid is above eighteen years of age, fine, legally, they are now adults, but that does not mean that they can make all decisions of their life independently. The parents should continue to have a say in their affairs until they are much older."

She told me the whole story.

"But your son was trying to do such a noble deed. Why did you have a problem with that?" I asked.

"Are you kidding me? Maybe you don't have children of your own. How would you feel if you sent your kids to school, and they convinced your child to do something that you do not agree with or do not believe in? How can I trust someone to inject something into my child? My child is perfectly fine and healthy. I wish health to all the other children in the world, but not at the expense of my child's health. We trust the doctors, but you cannot deny that in the name of research, a lot of dark things have happened in the past. Isn't it true that black people were injected with syphilis, and treatment was withheld all in the name of research? Isn't it true that American surgeons were performing surgeries on black female slaves without anesthesia, believing that black women do not suffer pain as if they were not human?" She made her point.

"What happened then? Did your son end up donating the cells?" I asked.

"We were new in the country. It is not easy being an immigrant, you see. We strictly told our son that he should not talk to that lady again, and there was absolutely no way I was going to let anyone inject something into my child and take blood from his body. But my son was being told that he had uneducated, unaware, and old-fashioned parents from a different country, and by not agreeing to donate cells, he was putting the life of another kid in jeopardy.

Our son did not want to upset us, but on the other hand, he was having feelings of extreme guilt for denying his blood to someone in need. He left home for a few weeks and was living with a friend. He succumbed to the pressure and eventually donated his blood cells without our consent. At school, they told him that he did not need our consent. This brought about such a big rift in our family that we still have not recovered from it. After a few weeks, when he wanted to come back home, his father gave him resistance and told him why he was coming back home if he would not listen to his parents.

Our family was put through a major torment because of people like you. You come and ask young adults to participate in your donation program, but you don't care about the views of their families. In our opinion, what you are doing is shameful and sinful."

She expressed her inner feelings without any hindrance.

"I can fully understand what you are talking about. And yes, I agree that I will never want my children to do anything against my will if I think that they are making a wrong decision. But here I would like to tell you that based on my understanding, this is a perfectly safe procedure and gives a new life to another person who would die otherwise. If one of my own children decided to become a bone marrow donor, I would fully support that. Your children are like my own children to me. If I felt that there was even an ounce of danger or threat to you or your children by becoming bone marrow donors, I would not be conducting this bone marrow donation drive," I put my point of view in front of her.

After the conversation ended, the couple went inside the mosque to pray. I turned around and saw a few kids who looked like they were in their late teens gathered and sent over by Ahmet to sign up as donors. They were ready to put their information on the signup sheet, having no clue about what they were doing and not understanding the depth of decision-making.

Quite shaken by the conversation I had with the Turkish couple earlier; I told the kids to take the pamphlets home and discuss them with their parents before signing up. I packed up my materials, ended the drive for that day, and proceeded to the mosque for prayers.

I realized that things were not as simple as they seemed to me. For my level of understanding of the topic, I was entirely clear about what the right thing to do was.

But for people who had a very limited understanding of the topic and all the myths, mistrusts, and misunderstandings prevalent in society, I was too naive to think that I would just show up and have people sign up as donors and it would be a simple task.

This required much more than that. This required educating the masses and taking steps toward allaying the anxieties and mistrust that people had in the medical profession. This required systemic debunking of conspiracy theories.

Gifts from a dying man

A few weeks ago, when I was on hematology service, I got a call about Mack, who was a twenty-eight-year-old man who was admitted to the trauma intensive care unit.

It was, unfortunately, another one of those tragic motorcycle accidents. We were called because his platelets were too low.

My residents and fellows saw and presented the case to me. We thought that there wasn't much for us to offer, and the low platelets were likely due to multiple aspects of his critical condition.

The ICU team had been trying to extubate him, but it looked like all efforts were failing, and the ICU attending had been called to evaluate for brain death. We, as a hematology team, went to the ICU.

The family visiting room was right outside the ICU unit. As we passed by, we heard loud wails and sobs from the room. He was a handsome young man who worked as a firefighter at the local fire department.

He had multiple hobbies, and riding and fixing motorcycles was one of them. Apparently, he was going at a very slow speed and was known to be a careful rider, but a big truck hit him at an intersection.

He was wearing full protective gear and his helmet, too, but the impact of the trauma was so hard that it ruptured his spinal cord and also caused significant brain injury.

He had three kids who were still in elementary school, and apparently, he was on his way to join the rest of the family to attend his daughter's piano recital.

We entered the patient's room. At least a dozen infusions were hanging by his bedside, including pressors, antibiotics, and fluids.

He was on a ventilator, and his whole body was swollen with the amount of fluids that had already been pumped into his veins. His pupils were not reacting to the light shown into them. He wasn't gagging when the endotracheal tube was pushed further into his throat.

There was a woman wearing scrubs standing by his bedside, entering some data into the computer.

"Hi, we are the hematology team. Is it OK if we examine him?" I asked.

"Oh, sure. I am from the Organ Procurement Organization. He had signed up as an organ donor, and as soon as the ICU attending declares him brain dead, our team will arrive to take him to the OR to procure his organs. I have already talked to the family, and they are all in agreement.

They are planning an open casket funeral, so our surgical team will make sure the body is prepared for that," she explained.

Although Mack was in the process of leaving this world with a widow and three orphans, while doing so, he was giving life to multiple people who were otherwise dying because of failed organs. He was about to win the prayers and gratitude of a number of dying patients and their families.

While the tree of his life was being uprooted and the harmony of his own family was being shattered, he was sowing the seeds of life into the gardens of several other families.

He was a hero.

While his own family was wailing in despair, several other families were smiling with teary eyes, about to receive some gifts from a dying man.

I turned around and asked the intern, who like myself, was also a foreign graduate, and asked her, "Have you thought about signing up as an organ donor?"

"I had never thought about it before, but the other day, as I was filling out the driver's license application form, it had that question, and I did not know what to say," she had responded.

"What did you end up doing then?" I asked.

"I checked off the box that said, 'Skip the question.'"

A Desi Wedding, Explained for my American Friends

I was recently in Peshawar to attend my younger brother's wedding. It was a long time, more than a decade since there was a wedding in my family, so everybody was excited, including myself.

After spending a week full of festivities and fun, when I came back to Rochester, all my American friends were excited to see the pictures and know the details of the wedding.

I think Bollywood has done an amazing job of portraying desi weddings to the world. (If desi is a new word for you, the dictionary meaning of this word is "of, from or characteristic of India, Pakistan or Bangladesh.")

There is no doubt that these weddings are some of the most fun domestic events carried out anywhere in the world. As I was showing the pictures and explaining traditions, I realized that I couldn't do justice to the descriptions in bits and pieces and there is a lot to tell so it would be nice to put some of the information together as an essay for those who like reading.

Wedding events can have some variations depending on the local region but there are three primary events that essentially all Pakistani weddings have. These are called the Mehndi, Baraat and Walima. These are the rough equivalents of Western weddings' rehearsal dinner, the wedding ceremony and reception, and the post- wedding brunch.

In days before these events, there might be smaller gatherings called 'Dholki's' (Urdu word for a small drum) where the closer family members and friends get together.

After the three main events, there are usually dinners or lunches hosted by close family members and the number of people that attend these after-events are smaller.

The first two main events that is the Mehndi and the Baraat are hosted by the bride's family and the Walima is hosted by the groom and his family.

The three events traditionally take place on consecutive days, but it is not uncommon for the events to be spaced apart by a day or two either to allow for rest or travel or some other reasons such as non-availability of wedding venues.

Mehndi

Mehndi is the Urdu translation of the word Henna. Henna is a plant/shrub, the leaves of which are crushed into a brown powder. A pasty version of this powder is used to either dye hair or apply to skin in various patterns that make great temporary tattoos.

This can be applied anywhere on the body but most commonly applied to the hands or feet in intricately beautiful designs.

This first event of the wedding is named as such because the groom along with his family goes to the bride's house and large, beautifully arranged trays of mehndi are brought along.

The girls apply mehndi to each other and also to the bride's hands and feet. The groom is brought in and sits right next to the bride and family members enjoy on the dance floor which is typically situated right in front of them.

This is the last night when the groom and bride will spend without each other. After this night, they are supposed to be together every night for the rest of their lives.

Baraat

This is the main event when the bride finally goes to the groom's house. Baraat is also called Rukhsati, which means Departure (of the bride from her father's home to the husband's.)

On this event, the groom goes, along with his family and friends in the form of a procession to the bride's house or to another venue where they may be hosting the event.

Typically, they all gather at the groom's house and then hop into their cars and go in a long queue together so that the passersby can tell that it's a wedding procession. Some people will also turn their hazard lights on to signal that they are part of the procession.

The groom's car is dolled up with flowers. In olden days, this procession used to go on horses which is not done that commonly anymore, but some people even today might arrange for the groom to enter the event venue on horseback.

Once the procession reaches the bride's house, the Nikah ceremony takes place which is a solemn event when the Maulana (priest) recites the religious prayers and officially weds the two.

Unlike in western weddings, there is no declaration by the priest for the groom to kiss the bride because public displays of physical affection are considered unacceptable in the society.

After some dancing and a lavish meal, the bride says a teary goodbye to her family and goes to the groom's house along with the procession.

Walima

This is an event hosted by the groom and his family. The marriage has already taken place by this time and the bride and groom are now together in hosting their guests.

Since the previous two events are hosted by the bride's family, this now is a chance for the groom to invite any guests that are closer to the latter family. This is a relatively simple event compared to the previous two.

A common tradition is for the groom's friends to ask the groom if the Walima is a "true" Walima or not. Those are code words to ask if they had sex on the night of the baraat or not. If the groom says Yes, then everybody rejoices.

If the groom says No, then everybody tries to troubleshoot the reason which can range from the bride not feeling well to maybe being on her menstrual cycle or the groom may have some difficulty performing.

If the groom is too shy or private to answer such a question, then people guess whether the Walima is "true" or not by his body language and whether he is appearing happy and joyful versus edgy, irritable and unfulfilled.

At different times during the main events, there are a number of traditions that are followed. These local traditions may vary depending on the region but I'm sure that you would enjoy reading about some of these.

"Drink some milk if you want to get married next"

This tradition typically takes place when the bride comes to the groom's house for the first time as the Baraat procession brings her from her father's house. She is given a glass of milk to take a sip from. The milk is mixed with nuts and honey, nicely warmed up and is truly delicious. She hands over the glass to the groom who also takes a sip. The glass of milk is now considered to have transformed into a potion that whoever drinks, will get married soon.

The men who are either the same age as the groom or younger, who are still unmarried, jump forward to get hold of the glass and take a few sips.

The younger boys, who have hit puberty but are still too shy about getting married, nervously refuse the drink.

The girls do not even take a look because a girl would look too "forward" if she openly declared that she wants to get married.

The older men stand around joking about how they are fed up with their spouses and how they should also take a sip and maybe it will open a new door for them too.

Someone joked that I should take a sip but after a marriage gone sour, I decided to stay away from the sweet poison for as long as I could.

This tradition is very similar to the "Bouquet Toss" in a western wedding where the bride throws a bouquet over her shoulder and amongst the single bridesmaids, whoever catches it, gets the good omen of finding love and getting married next.

As a bridesmaid, you are thinking that if it still doesn't work for you and you still don't get married, it's still a good idea to try to catch it if you want to go home with a beautiful bouquet.

The Act of Throwing Money

At any of these events, there is always loud music. This is either a live band or more commonly, a DJ is hired who brings in all his equipment including loudspeakers and the mixer.

The DJ's staff carry with them a large amount of cash. These are all in small bills stacked and stapled together. Each small bill carries the value, let's say of a dollar bill (not in terms of the actual stock exchange rate but rather in terms of the local "spending power" value of the money.) Right in front of the music setup is a clear area, which is made into a dance floor.

The dance floor gets particularly busy at different moments during the event such as when the Mehndi trays are brought in or when the groom walks in for the first time accompanied by the groomsmen.

This is when you have to buy some stacks of small bills (notes) and throw them in the air on top of the groom or other people who are dancing.

There is a variety of ways in which the notes can be thrown with dexterity and some people particularly show off their money throwing skills. The DJ's staff are very quick to bend down to the floor, the "note-pickers", and they keep collecting the money and putting it back into their cash reservoir.

This money ends up being a substantial portion of their earnings for the night and is loosely negotiated at the time of setting up the final rates for the job.

I had mixed feelings about this tradition. Since I have been living in America for the last two decades, I have been somewhat removed from the Pakistani wedding culture.

I spoke to my younger brother who routinely goes to these weddings and throws money generously and proudly. I told him how I felt that this tradition is hard for me to carry out because we have always been taught the respect of money.

Hard-earned money should not be thrown pompously like this when there might be people in the same neighborhood who are sleeping without having enough to feed their children.

Life has shown us well-off people lose their money, sometimes instantly. There is nothing as miserable as a rich person going poor.

I have not seen any other culture having a tradition of throwing money except for men throwing money at strippers in a strip club. My brother rebuked me for my thought process and told me that I was perhaps overthinking it.

He asked me to let a tradition remain a beautiful tradition and try not to put negative connotations to it. He told me that it is a way of showing your happiness and the tradition has been going on for, who knows how many centuries and whatever my pocket allows, I should partake in it.

Before the wedding, I had in my mind that I will not throw money. When the festivities began and people started dancing to loud music, the stage was set for close friends and family members to start throwing money.

I resisted for a while but then started feeling awkward that I was so close to the groom being his older brother and was not participating in one of the old traditions. This is when I also bought a stack of notes and started throwing the money at him.

To participate fully, I even handed over some cash to some of the teenagers for them to throw, thinking that if their parents did not like this practice, then I would be in trouble.

I thought to myself that this was an example of how difficult it is to stop yourself from doing what everybody else is doing even if you don't want to.

This "not doing" can sometimes be even more difficult than "doing" what other people are not doing. I was confused as to whether to act loyal to my culture and try to keep a tradition alive or to risk appearing "stuck up" by not following it since it went somewhat against my own principles.

"Give us money if you want to spend the night with your bride."

The night of the Baraat is the first night that the "just married" couple will spend together. Needless to say, that this is the most important night perhaps of their entire lives.

They are filled with excitement to finally be with each other and of course the prospect of making love for the first time. It doesn't come that easy though.

From the time they are sitting on the wedding stage, the bridesmaids start asking the bridegroom for money in order to let him take the bride to his home.

They traditionally also take away one of his shoes and do not give it back to him unless if he doles out some cash (Joota Chupai – "hiding of the shoe.")

There is haggling that goes on for quite a while and no amount seems to make the girls happy. The groom, already burdened by the expenses of the wedding, tries to shortchange them.

Once they agree on a certain amount, the girls finally give him back his shoe but to his consternation, when he brings her back home, the entry to the house is blocked by his own friends having the same demand.

Another long negotiating session takes place, and he gives the rest of his money to his friends to be able to finally spend some alone time with his new bride.

It doesn't end there though. As he is about to finally enter the wedding room, his own cousins and other youngsters in the family block his way to the bedroom.

His pockets already emptied out from previous encounters, now he turns to his friends to borrow some money to finally be left alone with his new wife.

If this tradition starts becoming too prolonged, some elders usually ask for it to be curtailed because it is usually already a late hour in the morning and the newly married couple often have to wake up at a decent time the next day for a festive brunch.

The crying bride

As I was showing some pictures of the Rukhsati (the departure) to some of my American friends, they were curiously asking why the bride and her close family members were crying when she was finally leaving for the groom's house at the end of the Baraat event.

This is because in Pakistani culture the girl lives at her father's house until she gets married. This is the moment when she is finally leaving that house and will now live in her husband's house.

This is also traditionally how a bride should be conducting herself on the night of the Baraat.

She should be putting on display her grief about leaving her father's home and should be hiding her excitement at getting married.

If she is appearing too playful, the aunties are quick to comment, "Look at today's brides, how inappropriate. Not shedding a single tear!" She has to find the right balance though.

If she sheds too many tears, it can spoil her expensive make-up that she spent a lot of time and money on, at the beauty salon.

In Western culture, a child after finishing high school wants to leave the parents' house and build a life of their own. It is considered a matter of pride for the child to leave the house and move towards adulthood. Even if desi parents living in the West want to follow their tradition and ask the kids to stay in their house, the teenagers start having a feeling of being losers if they are still living with their parents.

Nonetheless, whenever a child is finally leaving the parental home, it is a sad moment just like when a child is going to college after finishing high school, there are a lot of tears that are shed.

My daughter who is finishing high school in about a year is already talking about moving out for college. It feels so unfair to me that I only got to have her living with me for two decades of her life.

I often ask her to stay in our house and go to college locally, but she rightfully responds by telling me that I was the one always encouraging her to go wherever she wanted, to build whatever life and career she dreams of.

I know I will have to fight back my tears the day she leaves for college. As a Pakistani father, this day of being separated from my daughter would have come much later if I was in Pakistan, that is when she would have been married.

But now living here in the US, I will have to see this day much sooner. The bright side is that I will not be crying on her wedding day.

The Bed Jumps

This tradition is probably not very widely practiced in the country but more belongs to our local area. When the groom is brought in to see the bride on the day of the Baraat, a basic wooden bed is brought in. This is the kind of bed called a "Charpoy."

Since our country and region had been under British rule, if you open an Urdu dictionary, you will now see not an insignificant number of words that are derived from the English language.

But I have a suspicion that this word, as it is found in the Oxford Dictionary, has been taken by the English from Urdu. "Char" means four and "pai" means feet.

This is a simple bed with a wooden frame with ropes intertwined between the wooden sides. That makes it a "Charpai" (Four Feet.) The English word "Charpoy" is a derivation from that.

Here a charpai is brought in which is beautified with flowers and confetti. The groom is made to sit in the charpai, and the men surround it and lift it up and jump the groom up in the air along with the charpai.

My brother happens to be a man of size so the charpai was quite heavy to begin with. I went forward to lend a hand. You cannot stand back and just watch because it is a matter of showing that you are a tough man. Some other men also came forward.

As we gave the first jump, the bed swung and instead of going straight up, got lopsided. As we looked, that was the side held by all little kids who looked plenty in number but did not have much in terms of collective strength.

We quickly balanced the weight of the charpai amongst the adults and after just one or two jumps, the bed started getting heavier and heavier with each jump.

Our muscles started tiring quickly and I realized that the adults were withdrawing one by one. Now only I and a couple other guys were left lifting it up.

Finally, I yelled, "put it down!" while the surrounding people were screaming asking us to keep going on because they were having fun.

We still were able to put the groom back on the floor along with the charpai. I was relieved that the heavy work was over but then someone put a small kid on the charpai and we were expected to give him jumps too.

The same cycle repeated and now came to find out that no child wanted to be left behind. We kept at this tiresome for us but fun for others tradition. At the end of it, I had sweated under my fancy clothes and felt like I just finished a strenuous gym workout.

Other traditions may have some superstitious meaning behind them, but I still fail to understand the story behind this one except for the groomsmen having rowdy fun.

Sit a boy, in the bride's lap, so that she bears a boy

In this tradition, a young boy, usually a preteen, is made to sit in the lap of the bride. This is supposed to be a wish that the bride will have a son as her first child.

My American-born and raised kids were quick to point out the sexism and to express their shock at the inappropriateness of this tradition, in their eyes.

Now a lot of questions can be raised in today's world but there is no denying the fact that gender choice for children has remained a prevalent issue perhaps ever since humans have been around.

We still remain confused about gender issues and people differ vastly in their opinions about which traditions to rectify and what issues to accept and liberalize.

When my daughter asked me if this tradition should continue, I told her that I'm not the one to stop a tradition.

I can say whether I like it or not, but I cannot stop other people from thinking what they have been thinking for hundreds and thousands of years.

How a wedding feels in the days of social media and cell phones

One thing that was obvious was that it felt like every move was being made in order to be filmed and photographed. The photographers were constantly instructing everyone to pose here and there. It would often even come in the way of spontaneity.

For any of the traditions I described above, you had to wait for the cameraman's instructions. If you went too fast, you had to either slow down or even repeat a certain tradition.

Long pauses came in the middle of a certain ceremony or tradition if the lighting or standing arrangement was not to the standards of the cameraman.

It became annoying to the point that I suggested that the cameramen leave for about twenty minutes.

Enough memories had been captured on film, but we had not had any unfilmed moments where we all, as a family could just focus on each other and on enjoying ourselves at this time of merriment rather than being concerned about filming and how our pictures and videos will come out.

My request was instantly rejected by almost everyone because people liked it that way. They wanted to be filmed continuously and were more interested in the social media depiction of the event than enjoying the current moment.

I concluded in my mind that perhaps humans enjoy the new digital ways more than they enjoy living in the moment and there is no use fighting the new ways of the world.

Ever since humans have inhabited the Earth, there have been countless philosophies, religions and ways of living different aspects of life. These can all be very different from each other.

However, when it comes to how a man and a woman should live together, marriage is the only way that humans have come up with, as a legitimate practice in any society.

All countries, cultures and religions require men and women to be married in order to coexist respectfully. But it remains to be a tricky arrangement.

There is a famous desi saying that goes something like, "Marriage is like a sweet dessert – those who are eyeing it are salivating and those who have already eaten it are repenting."

Essays by a Divorced Single Dad

A Doctor and His Daughter on Becoming a Doctor

My grandfather could not read or write. Still not so unfortunate to be unable to send his children to school. He moved them from the village to the city and put them in a school.

Not only did he give his children the opportunity to learn but he also passed on to them the discipline to work hard and excel in school and go into competitive and respectable professions of Medicine and Law.

My father was a valedictorian and had a very successful career as a Pediatrician. My brothers and I followed suit and went into the same professions. Becoming a doctor came natural to me and I found it easy to navigate the already well-trodden path by my family.

As my own children are now growing up, I found it hard to know how much to guide them when it came to their own choice of career. Another level of complexity was added by the fact that I immigrated to America.

The practices of parents and how much influence they had on their children's career choices were very different compared to Pakistan where most parents insist that their kids choose between just a few professions, that is, becoming a Doctor, Lawyer, or an Engineer.

I am a proud parent in that my daughter Zaina graduated from high school and has entered college this year.

Over the years, I have had conversations with her regarding what she should do for a career when she grows up. As we move her out of the house into her college dorm room this month, I have put together a dialogue between her and myself that you will find interesting if you are a parent, or a child who has given any thought to "how to make a career choice."

This dialogue did not take place in one sitting but in bits and pieces over a number of years.

. . .

Me: So, what do you want to become when you grow up?

Zaina: I don't know (shrugging her shoulders.)

Me: I think you should start thinking about it. It will be one of the most important decisions of your life. What about your school friends? Have they started saying what they want to do for a living when they grow up?

Zaina: It's not something that we really talk about. But it's kind of a joke at school how brown and Asian parents are so overly focused on their kids' careers and apparently all brown parents want their children to become doctors. White parents on the other hand just let their kids do what they want to do, what they like to do.

Me: I totally get it that there is a difference amongst parenting styles. I remember that once I had asked one of my White colleagues what her daughter wanted to be when she grew up and she had said that she moved to California and wanted to become a dancer. Although there's nothing wrong with doing that, it was just ingrained in me that becoming a dancer cannot be a suitable career choice. So, I asked her, 'but what did you want her to be?' She turned around and gave me the kind of a look that you give someone when you don't like the question. 'Happy!' she responded in just one word.

Very different for brown parents though. There was a Russel Peters show where he was making a joke that if a brown kid growing up in America decides to become a doctor, that means that he or she does not have any independent thought process and is just following his parents' wishes blindly.

Zaina: The world is so full of interesting things to do and tremendous possibilities. Why is it that brown parents are stuck on making their kids into doctors and think that whatever else they do will be all doom and gloom?

Me: I think this is because of our own childhood. Where we grew up, it was very hard to make a good living in other professions. Getting into a medical school was a sort of a guarantee that you will be well-respected by the society, and you will earn a good living. In developing countries, if you don't earn well, your quality of life can be really bad. You may not even be able to afford some basics such as buy a house or have a decent car unless you have inherited some money. Yes, people in other professions also do quite well but financial success is not guaranteed.

Zaina: Well, that is not the case here in America. You can have a decent life in almost any profession. We are told in schools to follow our passions and not worry too much about how much money we will be making. You also don't want to end up making good money, but every day wake up to a job that you hate to do. Also, a lot of kids don't want to put in so much time and effort into such prolonged studies. You have to be in school for so long to become a doctor.

Me: Those are great points and that is exactly why we are having this conversation. As a parent, it is hard to decide how much to be involved with your children in terms of guiding them towards the choice of a certain career. White parents can tend to be too "hands off" and let the kids make their own decisions where they should provide some guidance because how mature can a kid's mind be at high school age. Some Asian parents on the other hand can be viewed as "helicopter" parents and be too overbearing and demanding their kids to adopt certain career choices fulfilling their own dreams rather than letting the kids pursue their passions.

Zaina: So, what are you saying?

Me: I'm saying that you are growing into a very smart young woman and whatever decision you make will be a good one. But I can at least tell you that whatever you choose to do, if the career of your choice fulfills four criteria, I will think that you chose a great profession.

Zaina: And what are those four criteria?

Me: A career should be financially rewarding, intellectually stimulating, socially giving and personally forgiving.

Zaina: Woo, that is a mouthful. Now you have to tell me what you mean by that.

Me: Well, first of all, nobody can deny that the biggest reality of life is money. When you put all your effort into doing something it is only fair that you should be paid well. If all your life, you are struggling to juggle your finances and are not able to provide adequately for yourself and your family, not only do you suffer in day-to-day living, but you are also not able to engage in more pleasurable things in life. You are always trying to make ends meet.

Look at the example of teachers. They are the most important workers of any society. They build a society. But their wages are very low compared to so many other professions. You know how they say that if you are made the President of the country for one day, what would you do? I usually say that I will make teachers the highest-paid people in society and then see how everybody will be flocking to become a teacher.

Even different sciences pay differently. I have a friend whose dream was to become a marine biologist. After going to college for a few years he realized that although he would be living his dream, he would not be able to afford all his groceries easily, so he changed paths and became a radiation oncologist. He wished that someone had told him earlier about the income potential of different jobs rather than being told only to pursue his passions. A kid should be forewarned if his or her passion doesn't pay well.

It is so common for kids to go to college, take huge loans to pursue degrees of their choice, and graduate to find out that their jobs barely pay enough to manage their daily expenses let alone pay off the loans quickly and easily. A philosophy professor may be the highest educated person in society but might make less in a year than what is needed to live a comfortable life.

Zaina: That all makes sense, but the problem is that brown parents care about nothing else. They just want their kids to become money-making machines. There is more to life than just worrying about how to make money. It is probably equally worse to be stuck in doing what you don't like to do in order to make good money as compared to being stuck with what you like to do but not being able to make a good living.

Me: You are right! That brings me to the second criterion. Whatever you do should be intellectually stimulating.

Zaina: Now what is that all about?

Me: What makes humans superior to all other forms of life on this planet is our brains. We share all our other functions with animals but since we have the ability to think and have higher intelligence, we claim superiority over all other species. Now within the human species, it's the same thing that makes certain people superior to others. Intellect. Whoever uses their intelligence the most is regarded the most in a society.

Zaina: But by that criterion, only academicians would be respected by society but if someone is not inclined that way and genuinely not interested in books, should they force themselves to study? That simply doesn't attract some people.

Me: Intelligence does not come only from books. Yes, it's true that if you are studying a subject formally and have done a lot of research or published many papers, it is highly regarded but you could be in a profession where the expertise might not come just from reading books. You should strive to be the best at what you are doing by using your brain. For example, if you sell flowers, you should strive to become the florist who knows the most about flowers! The quality of your flowers should be the best. You should make the best bouquets. Not only should you try to be good at the business of selling flowers, but you should use your intellect to dive deep into the study of flowers to the point that your knowledge should put a Botanist or a Floriculturist to shame.

Zaina: So basically, what you are saying is not to just focus on making a living but to try to become the best at what you do by using your intellect to become an expert at your trade.

Me: You got it.

Zaina: But is that necessary? If you have a business that is bringing you tons of money, why can't you just enjoy life and not worry too much about becoming the most knowledgeable person in that field?

Me: Yes, you can do that but that makes for a shallow personality. You will see people in your life who inherit a fortune, and they do not have to work at all. They have more money than their multiple generations can spend. They can live a hedonistic life but that lacks any sense of achievement or self -actualization. If a person, who is not financially dependent on his or her income, becomes an expert in a certain trade, their respect goes to an entirely different level.

Zaina: Yes, I know what you mean. There is a girl in our school whose parents are apparently so wealthy that they live like the royals. She doesn't even need to go to school but she spends the most time studying because she wants to join NASA and become an astronaut. No wonder she is so popular. Anyways, what else should I look for in a job?

Me: Oh, the third criterion! Whatever you do for a living should be socially giving.

Zaina: Socially giving! Now what does that mean?

Me: It means that whatever you are doing, if you are also helping people, preferably without charging them for it, you will find it to be the most satisfying. My dad was a pediatrician. In his private practice, he would see a lot of poor people. Every time he sensed that a patient or their family was struggling to pay his fees, he would waive it off. I know restaurant owners who routinely feed hungry people without charging them. I know several lawyers who work pro bono even if they don't have to. This is the essence of being a good human being. Using your skills to help people and not focus just on making your own living.

Zaina: In a way, aren't you helping people no matter what you do? Any time you are providing service to someone; you are helping them right?

Me: Well, there are some jobs where you are only helping privileged people get more privileged. For example, if you are an investment banker who takes on clients who have let's say, a minimum of a million dollars to invest, you are helping the rich get richer. If you are a luxury yacht dealer, you are helping to further elevate the already extravagant lifestyle of your customer. There is absolutely nothing wrong with those occupations but at the end of the day, you have not helped a person in misery or at the time of need. If you still want to give back to the society, you can donate money, but you will not have the gratification that one achieves by giving hands-on help to someone.

Zaina: Yes, I can see that.

Me: That brings me to my last criterion. Make sure that the career you are choosing is personally forgiving.

Zaina: Personally forgiving! What does that mean?

Me: It means that whatever you end up doing in life, make sure that your job does not consume your entire existence. Leave some space, in fact a lot of space, to do things outside of your occupation. You will be surprised to see that this balance can be very hard to achieve.

I remember once going to an annual gala put together by the local Academy of Medicine. There was an awards ceremony and after dozens of people came to the podium to receive their awards, they announced the final award which was some sort of a lifetime achievement award given to a physician-scientist who had made extraordinary discoveries in his lab. After accepting his award, he first pointed towards a group of people in the audience and asked them to stand up. He introduced them as his "work family," that is, his co-workers from his lab. He thanked them and told the audience how he could not have achieved what he did without their help. Then he pointed towards another small group of people in the audience and had them stand up. These were his family members including his wife, children and grandkids. Instead of thanking them, he apologized to them publicly for how absent he was in his home life. He admitted to being a failure in all his personal relationships because he was so consumed by the passion of his job. Everybody could see the disdain on the faces of the family members accentuated by the tears in his wife's eyes.

Zaina: Yes, I would not want to be in that situation.

Me: There are other examples. I see cancer patients all the time who have a similar story. They work all their lives thinking of traveling or pursuing hobbies when it's time for their retirement but get diagnosed with serious illness just within a few months of retiring. I used to moonlight at a hospital and whenever I needed to obtain a gastroenterology consult, there was this one consultant who was always working. Even on weekends and long holidays. After a break of a few months, I was on the floor looking up his number but couldn't find it, so I asked a nurse for his contact information. She looked at me and replied, 'Oh you don't know he died? In fact, he was working in the hospital one weekend and he collapsed on the floor. They called a code blue, but they could not revive him. He came to work in the morning and was taken to the morgue by the afternoon.'

Zaina: Oh boy! That did not end too well. So, in a nutshell you are telling me to find a career that is financially rewarding, intellectually stimulating, socially giving and personally forgiving... Is that your way of being a brown dad and convincing me to become a doctor?

Me: Well. It's up to you how you take this advice but whatever you end up doing, try to beat that! I would love you and support you in whatever you do. And make sure you are not just fulfilling some criteria but are also happy with your choice.

I Heard you got Divorced, Congratulations!

Two women in their thirties meet unexpectedly at a gathering and realize that they are seeing each other after fifteen years. The last time they spent time together was when they were in high school. Then the paths of their lives diverged, and they did not keep in touch. Now was a good time to catch up. Their names are "Unhappily Married" and "Happily Divorced." The following dialogue ensues:

UNHAPPILY MARRIED: God, I can't believe running into you like this. So nice to see you after such a long time. How's life treating you?

HAPPILY DIVORCED: Life is great. I have no complaints. Tell me how your parents are? I can still remember spending the long afternoons at your house during summer break. Your mom used to make the best lemonade. How is she? How is your dad?

UNHAPPILY MARRIED: My mom is doing great. She has some health issues now and can't take care of things like she used to, but we take good care of her.

HAPPILY DIVORCED: And your dad?

UNHAPPILY MARRIED: He passed away two years ago. Sudden, massive heart attack. Wasn't even alive when the ambulance came.

HAPPILY DIVORCED: Oh I'm so sorry to hear that (eyes welling up.) I can't believe it! That's so sad. He wasn't even that old? And he was always physically so fit?

UNHAPPILY MARRIED: Yes, I know. None of us saw it coming. It still feels like yesterday.

HAPPILY DIVORCED: How's your husband? And kids?

UNHAPPILY MARRIED: Oh we are okay. My husband got a promotion. He isn't home a lot. But that can be a good thing. The kids are doing well at school. Sara is now in high school; can you believe it? And Adam is now in seventh grade.

HAPPILY DIVORCED: I remember them being so little! I have such a cute picture of both of them that I have framed. You need to come visit us sometime very soon.

UNHAPPILY MARRIED: I know. I'm just so happy to see you again. You tell me. How are your husband and kids doing?

HAPPILY DIVORCED: We are doing amazing. Actually we got divorced last year and are currently sharing custody of our kids.

UNHAPPILY MARRIED: Oh my God, I'm so sorry to hear that. I didn't even know! How awful! My heart is breaking! How did that happen?

HAPPILY DIVORCED: Actually this is not a sad life event for me so I would rather that you congratulate me rather than commiserate…

UNHAPPILY MARRIED: Oh I'm sorry, I know it can be very traumatic, and this is your way of coping but really, I'm sorry.

HAPPILY DIVORCED: No really! I'm very happy and getting divorced was as happy of an event for me as the birth of my kids or my graduation from college.

UNHAPPILY MARRIED: That's a very odd way of looking at it. I have never heard anyone congratulate anyone for being divorced. It is always thought of as a tragedy.

HAPPILY DIVORCED: That's true. I always used to think that way too. Until it happened to me. I realized how important a divorce can be for some situations. It can be a blessing and an event to rejoice for many.

UNHAPPILY MARRIED: Well I can understand your point but it's still very tragic. After all, a house gets broken. A family gets shattered.

HAPPILY DIVORCED: Yes, that happens but it's not always a time for all remorse. You have to look at the bright side. Just like anything else in life.

UNHAPPILY MARRIED: I'm still not so sure about that.

HAPPILY DIVORCED: Well let me ask you this. You remember when your grandma used to live with you? Remember how sick and debilitated she got towards the end? She had cancer for the longest time, and she was in extreme pain and misery and your family could not see her like that? When she finally died, you had secretly told me how everyone was sad for her to go but relieved internally that her misery ended. From that view, it was a happy moment in a way that you had wished would come sooner.

UNHAPPILY MARRIED: Yes, I do remember, and, in that sense, I agree that all of us were waiting for her suffering to end. Some things just don't come out right even if you try to put them into words tactfully. Some things are actually best left unsaid.

HAPPILY DIVORCED: I know but some thoughts should be shared with those who are closest to you. If you don't, they lead to a buildup of negative emotions in your head.

UNHAPPILY MARRIED: OK well thanks for sharing your true emotion with me. I knew that although I'm guilty of not remaining in touch, but you were always the kind of a friend who I knew that if I met even after a hundred years, it would feel as if I could share anything with you.

HAPPILY DIVORCED: Thanks and I feel the same about you.

UNHAPPILY MARRIED: So what actually happened? Why did you guys break up?

HAPPILY DIVORCED: Where do I start?

UNHAPPILY MARRIED: I know but something major must have happened?

HAPPILY DIVORCED: Let's just say that we didn't get along.

UNHAPPILY MARRIED: Isn't that true for a lot of marriages though?

HAPPILY DIVORCED: Yes, it is but sometimes the differences become too strong and unacceptable.

UNHAPPILY MARRIED: Well isn't that what marriage is about? It's a compromise. No couple is perfect. You have to learn how to live with your partner and have mutual respect.

HAPPILY DIVORCED: People who divorce understand that concept. But it's not always possible for two individuals to achieve that state of compromise. Do you think that people who end up being divorced don't try to compromise?

UNHAPPILY MARRIED: Yes, but it's a lifelong struggle. For some it's easy, for others it's difficult. But you have to keep trying. That is what marriage is all about. You have to put in a lot of effort to live happily ever-after.

HAPPILY DIVORCED: For some people, life doesn't roll like a fairy tale.

UNHAPPILY MARRIED: Who said every marriage is like a fairy tale. There are issues and struggles in every marriage.

HAPPILY DIVORCED: I feel that every time someone tries to enlighten me with the "marriage is a compromise between two individuals" idea, they are implying that this concept is somehow alien to people who get divorced. Some differences become uncompromisable, wait, is that even a word?

UNHAPPILY MARRIED: Actually I don't blame you. I can totally understand why something like that could happen to you. You had an arranged marriage. How can you marry someone who you don't even know. It's very obvious that if you don't know the personality of another person and are forced to marry them, it will not work normally.

HAPPILY DIVORCED: Well if that is a valid reason for divorce, then arranged marriages generally would not be so successful. But we all know that the rate of divorce is very low in places where there are more arranged marriages.

UNHAPPILY MARRIED: Yes, but the rate of living unhappily for the rest of your life, stuck with a person who you don't get along with is equally high in those apparently intact marriages.

HAPPILY DIVORCED: You are right. In the West, there are seldom any arranged marriages, but the divorce rate almost approaches fifty percent. That is a flip of a coin. It means that there is a fifty-fifty chance of you getting divorced. Isn't it crazy? But after having gone through divorce myself, I can tell you that a marriage being "arranged" by family versus getting married by falling in "love" has nothing to do with your happiness after you get married.

UNHAPPILY MARRIED: How can you say that?

HAPPILY DIVORCED: The critics of "arranged" marriages often mistake these marriages for forced marriages, which they are actually not. Matchmaking has been around since forever. If you research marriage, you will come to find out that this is one of the most enduring practices of humankind since the beginning of time. Humans have not yet found a superior and more acceptable arrangement for a man and woman to live together and procreate.

UNHAPPILY MARRIED: Interesting view.

HAPPILY DIVORCED: I actually read some books about the history of marriage after I got divorced. Trying to figure out where I went wrong.

UNHAPPILY MARRIED: Maybe you should have read those books before getting divorced! Just kidding.

HAPPILY DIVORCED: No but seriously, I found out that the concept of falling in love to get married to a person for the rest of your life is a relatively recent concept over the last few centuries. Marriages were not always like that. It was always sort of a contract between a man and a woman being assigned certain roles in life which both were happy with. It was supposed to be a symbiotic relationship with well-defined duties and responsibilities along with rights and perks. Somehow somewhere, the roles started blending and we were sold this idea that all marriages should be based on nothing else but love and if you marry the person who you fall in love with would be some sort of a guarantee that you will remain happy ever after. But guess what?

UNHAPPILY MARRIED: What?

HAPPILY DIVORCED: That narrative totally misses the point that humans can fall out of love as commonly and easily as they can fall into love. Sometimes you don't have any control over it. Your mind keeps telling you that you are still supposed to love the person who you are married to, but your heart has fallen out of love. You don't have any control over it. Then you have to live the rest of your life with a person who you do not love anymore. That's where the "compromise" word comes into play!

UNHAPPILY MARRIED: I think you may have hit the nail in the head. I have not said this to anyone but since I have known you for so long, I know that you can keep a secret. What you are describing is exactly what I'm going through.

HAPPILY DIVORCED: Listen please don't get me wrong. I wasn't really talking about you. I'm sorry if I…

UNHAPPILY MARRIED: No you didn't say anything wrong. I'm just telling you that we have been married for twelve years now. I don't love him the same way as I used to when we initially got together. And I know that he keeps telling me that he loves me every now and then but deep inside I know that he has lost the spark too. We say "I love you" to each other when we have to. But it doesn't come to our lips as naturally as it used to. It can be an effort to say that at times.

HAPPILY DIVORCED: But you guys look so good together. Always smiling and looking so good as a couple. I follow your Instagram profile and the parties that you host, the fun times you guys have as a family, the vacations that you take... We are always talking about how you guys have a perfect marriage.

UNHAPPILY MARRIED: I know. We are happy in that way. God has given us more than we could ever ask for. He still respects me and gives me my space. He is a great father. He is so good to my family. But he somehow is not the same person that I married. There is no warmth in him towards me anymore. I could see it in his eyes, in his touch. Now even his hugs have become very cold. The sex that was so passionate and soul-fulfilling, is as if it's a duty. Both of us are happy to stay away from it and often when one of us initiates it, the other feels like when you have to eat when at the dinner table but not wanting to eat from a full stomach.

HAPPILY DIVORCED: But does that matter? If you have your family intact and you are giving a loving home to your kids and have a respectable place in the society, you are succeeding in your marriage. Love becomes a secondhand emotion in this situation. Something you can live without when all the other needs are being fulfilled.

UNHAPPILY MARRIED: Yes, but that was not the only reason why we got married in the first place. Plus, it's hard to live like that. I wish that he could love me like he used to again but then I think why should I expect him to do that if I don't have those feelings towards him anymore.

HAPPILY DIVORCED: If it's that bad, then why don't you guys talk about it and get separated?

UNHAPPILY MARRIED: We have talked a little bit about it and us both kind of know how we feel towards each other. But we cannot even think about divorce. How could we do this to our children? They deserve to be raised in a loving household. Our parents and families would get devastated if we decided to get divorced. We would not have any place in the society. It would be a nightmare.

HAPPILY DIVORCED: I know the feeling. We lived like that for several years before we finally got divorced. Anytime one of us would even bring up the topic of being separated, it was filled with feelings of guilt. How could we put our own happiness above the need to give the kids an intact and loving home. How could you tear apart your own nest after having put it together, twig by twig, over so many years? It's not easy to destroy something that you have built yourself, with so much love.

UNHAPPILY MARRIED: I can understand the feeling.

HAPPILY DIVORCED: I used to look around me. All these couples around me. A lot of couples were having difficulty in their marriages. To me it almost looked like out of ten marriages, only two were happy. One where the couple was truly happy, head over heels in love with each other, perfect harmony. Another which was so bad that it ended in divorce very quickly. But the rest of the eight marriages, although intact, were mere "compromises" where the love was either lost or not there to begin with, but the marriage remained intact because that was the right thing to do.

UNHAPPILY MARRIED: How did your marriage break then? If you were ready for that compromise and were not selfish to break your home for your own happiness, how did it come to a point when you guys decided to divorce?

HAPPILY DIVORCED: Not everybody gets that lucky. Many people are living miserable lives, stuck with each other where they really don't want to, but don't have a way out. Sometimes things go so bad, and circumstances become so unpleasant and intolerable, that you have to part ways which is a blessing in disguise. If love is lost, that is still something you can live with, but when respect is lost and malice creeps in, then its best to get separated.

UNHAPPILY MARRIED: I wouldn't argue with that. But it's still sad for the children. If it weren't for the children, many people would have ended their marriages much sooner, including me!

HAPPILY DIVORCED: I think that is also another myth that needs to be broken. Who says that divorce is always bad for the kids? If it is, in what way is it bad for the children? Oftentimes it's better for them to have two separate loving parents than living under the same roof with two constantly fighting and antagonizing parents. There are many famous and successful men and women in history who were children of either single or divorced parents. For every child, that has had any problems in life due to being in a divorced household, I can show you ten children who have similar or even worse problems despite coming from intact but unhappy families.

UNHAPPILY MARRIED: Are you suggesting that I also get separated from my husband then?

HAPPILY DIVORCED: See that's a knee-jerk reaction that everybody gives me when I say things in support for divorce. By no means am I suggesting that you break your family apart but the point that I'm making is that divorce can actually be good for some situations and for some couples. Usually we spend too much time in misery before we are relieved of it. I want people to understand and be more accepting of this as a good solution to many problems rather than considering it as a negative life event at all times.

UNHAPPILY MARRIED: Okay I get your point. But tell me, what was he doing? Was he physically abusing you? He must be cheating on you right?

HAPPILY DIVORCED: Why should it matter to know the exact reason why a couple gets divorced? Isn't it enough to know that two people did not get along. I have seen that the story is very similar in all cases of divorce. It is very natural to think of the person that is closer to you as the victim and the other person to be the one at fault. Every man is accused of cheating, beating his wife, financially crippling the wife if in a male-earning relationship, drug abuser, raging alcoholic and unloving father. Every woman is accused of being lazy, spendthrift, having mental health issues and trying to alienate her husband from his friends and family. I have not seen the word "narcissist" used with so much consistency than to describe an ex-spouse. The irony is that this is the person who was considered so perfect in many ways that one was ready to spend the rest of one's life with. This is also the person who when described by close family or friends, is considered an amazing person in all other roles and relationships.

UNHAPPILY MARRIED: I can see that...

HAPPILY DIVORCED: At the end of the day, it doesn't really matter what led to the divorce or whose fault it was. It should be no surprise to people that it is perfectly understandable for two people not to get along to a point that they eventually decide to part ways which may seem to be against the commonly held wisdom of staying together to keep the family intact.

UNHAPPILY MARRIED: I have noticed some couples where one partner wants to divorce the other, but the other one wants to stay in the marriage.

HAPPILY DIVORCED: That is actually not uncommon at all, but you always have to see who eventually asked for the divorce. The person who asks for it is the one who wants out. He or she has had it so bad that they don't care about staying in the relationship anymore. They feel their freedom after the divorce. It's hard on the other party in the beginning but things settle down after a while for both.

UNHAPPILY MARRIED: How do you feel about getting married again?

HAPPILY DIVORCED: Ah, that is called the triumph of hope over experience!

UNHAPPILY MARRIED: (chuckles)

HAPPILY DIVORCED: I have seen many second marriages work much better. Probably because you have had time to think about your own deficiencies from your experiences and trying to rectify them in a future marriage. Also the expectations are much lower in a second marriage. You are happy if your spouse is not being negative and coexisting peacefully which is worth a lot more than constantly agonizing over the small things that they are not doing to prove their love to you. You become more forgiving and less demanding yourself.

UNHAPPILY MARRIED: Well I hope that you find a companion again one day. But be careful while you are promoting divorce in this way. It doesn't sit well with society if you talk that way.

HAPPILY DIVORCED: When has society liked anyone who points fingers towards flaws in the social structure. But if nobody does that, then how do you bring improvement in people's lives? Plus, divorce is not all fun and pleasure. There are many aspects of divorce that are uglier than staying in an unhappy marriage. But if you ever see two people really struggling with their marriage and if a relationship has been irreparably broken, it is better to facilitate an amicable divorce rather than trying to keep the marriage intact. That is the biggest gift for that family.

UNHAPPILY MARRIED: Well I understand your perspective. I know it's sad and tragic on one level but on another level a positive life event for some. I wish that your marriage had worked but if you put your all into it and it still didn't work out for you, I am happy for you now that you don't have to live that misery every single day of your life. Congratulations.

Please Let Me Have Lunch With My Child

A few weeks ago, we packed our bags, sat in a car, drove to another city, got keys to an apartment and settled my daughter in her new room. The next day we drove back home. She did not return with us. This was the first time in her life that she would spend a night on her own.

This was also the first time in my life that she would not be sleeping at home. And just like that. She was gone.

Life goes through many different phases. At different times you have different lives. The phases change every few years. They have to come and go. You don't have any control over it. You have to accept each new phase. The better you are at adapting to new phases, the happier you are.

Nobody's life is stuck in the same phase forever. Oftentimes the phases change either with the addition of a new person in your life or when somebody goes away.

Every phase brings with it some joys and some issues of sadness. Some phases have more joy. Others have more sadness. But you have to find joy in the sad times and remember your sad times during times of joy. The phases sometimes are predictable but other times change without any warnings or premonitions.

As I look back at my own life, I can still remember all the phases. There was a time when we were kids. This was the house of my childhood, where I had consciousness as a child. There were three of us brothers and we used to live with our stay-at-home mom.

At that age that was our whole world and as a child one could not even imagine that life will be different some day. We used to wake up in the morning and have breakfast as a family.

Our dad was a young doctor with a lot of working hours. He would himself drop us off at school. We would often be about ten minutes late to school and had to run around the school grounds a couple of times as punishment.

Our dad used to pick us up and we would have lunch together sometimes indoors but when the weather was good, at the patio garden. He would take a nap and then go to work in the evening.

We would just play in the yard or do our homework. Sometimes we would play with our neighbors. If someone were to invite us to a birthday party, we often could not go because we had only one car that my father used to go to work.

Also our mom didn't drive. She used to cook and clean and yell at us for not keeping things clean and tidy. We would always have dinner when our dad would come home. Then we used to go to sleep often, all three of us in the same room with the air conditioner on in the hot Peshawar summer.

The next phase I remember is when we were a bit older in the high school and college age. My younger brothers were born who were about eight to ten years younger than me. We did not have a sister, and it was just a lot of boys hanging out in the house doing boy stuff. Chasing each other, often fighting, laughing, watching movies and video games.

Our dad was older in his fifties and was at a much senior level at his job. We now had a driver who would drive us back and forth to school.

Our mom always allowed us to invite our friends over and oftentimes when friends of multiple brothers were over, the house would look like a dorm with boys of different ages roaming around.

A lot of our friends still tell us how they remember the moments spent at our house and we give credit to our mom to be gracious enough to host all these boys.

Later when we became parents ourselves, we realized that it was not an easy thing to do to control so many boys. I would always be fooling around with my two younger brothers following me wherever I went. Their job was to laugh at my jokes and do everything that I say. I was their big brother after all.

Then came the first time that I realized that you could also lose someone you love and that is how you can enter into the next phase of your life almost instantly.

My older brother had finished his medical college studies and had passed his exams to go to the United Kingdom for his postgraduate medical studies.

Over multiple dinner discussions, I knew that the overall plan was for him to go for a few years and then come back to take over our father's busy pediatrics practice.

It seemed like it would just be some training for a few years and then he would be back, and our lives would return to the same as they were. But then just like that, we drove him to the airport, waved him goodbye and then he was gone.

This was the first time it hit me that somebody that you love can go away from your life.

Yes, they are still there, and you can pick up the phone and talk to them any time. Yes, you can plan a trip and go meet them any time. Yes, they will come to visit you, and you will still get together for a lot of family gatherings.

But you will no longer wake up in the morning and see their uncombed hair. You will no longer be fighting over who finished the ice cream. You will no longer be sitting with that person in the same room for hours and not even talk to each other.

Since the day my brother left about thirty years ago, he started his own new life, and I did mine. We are always there for each other, but that phase of our life was over when we were living together, as elder brothers to our younger brothers and as teenage kids to our parents, all living under the same roof.

The phase that followed took several different shapes with a lot of changes in my life. This included leaving my house to come to America to build a career. This was the phase of independence and adventure.

It was a good feeling to be out in a different country experiencing a different way of life and a different culture. There were a lot of internships and random rotations in different hospitals. This included staying in temporary housing such as with friends or at hospital accommodations.

This included a yearlong jobless period and also a time when my visa was rejected in the aftermath of 9/11 when a lot of Muslim students from various countries were not being allowed easy access to jobs in the West. This same phase was filled with freedom and independence.

This was the time to go out in the world and try to make a name for yourself. I was so engrossed in myself and my own life and ambition that the thought did not even cross my mind that my parents and brothers might be missing me just like I was missing my older brother when he left home a few years ago.

This phase ended when I finally got a job. This was the time to settle down and begin my own family. I got a nice apartment in a very beautiful part of town. I got married and within a couple of years we had our first baby girl.

Three years later we had a baby boy and just like that we had a family of four. When kids are little, there is pretty much nothing else that you can accomplish. Rearing the kids is more than a full-time job.

We were in a foreign country and did not have any help from family. Most of our friends were in similar situations. Having been brought up in

Pakistan, both my wife and I had grown up with a lot of domestic workers in our houses but here we could not afford any hired help, just like everybody else.

I was also going through a medical residency where you are easily working eighty hours or more per week. There was literally nothing else on my mind other than work and kids.

In some ways, it was hard to manage but each smile and each kiss on the cheeks of the kids made any hardship easy to endure.

Around this time my father died which was one of my life's biggest losses but still since I was not living with him at that time, my day-to-day personal life did not change that much since I had left my father's home about a decade ago.

People say that the strongest love that you can have is towards your child.

Yes, we love our parents, our siblings and other family members. Yes, there is the romantic kind of love as well but that is slightly different. We are talking about love towards blood relatives.

But it is said that the love towards a child is even stronger than the love towards a parent. It may not be true for everyone, but most people will agree with that.

The way you get happy with your child's happiness and the way your heart is torn when your child is sad or hurt in any way can be compared to emotions towards anyone else, even towards your parents.

I have always had a theory behind this. Because our children are made from us biologically, we can feel their happiness and pain as if we feel our own emotions. Our parents feel the same way about us for the same reason. Our intensity of these emotions is not as high for our own parents because we are made from them, but they are not made from us.

An analogy would be that if your hand is hurt, you will also hurt because your hand is part of yourself. But the hand may not feel the pain if another part of your body is hurt such as the chest or the abdomen. The hand will feel it if one of your fingers is hurt because now the finger is a part of the hand.

When my kids were in elementary school, I was a very involved dad. I would not lose any opportunity to volunteer at their school.

Most of the volunteer activities were done by moms and a lot of times I would also feel a bit awkward in a room filled with kids, teachers and moms but I didn't care. I enjoyed being around my kids and their school lives so much that every few months I would try to get involved in some way.

My job was very demanding, and it was hard to take time off but once you set your mind to something, nothing is difficult. I would take a couple of hours away from work and go to the school to play my part.

One of these activities was to go and have lunch with my kids when they were in elementary school. I would find out what time the lunch period was. It was typically not more than just twenty minutes.

I would take time off from work about half an hour prior to that. I would reach the school and sign in to the visitors' book at the front office. They would usually give me a sticker that said "Visitor" that I would place on my lapel. I would go to the cafeteria and stand right outside the door of the cafeteria. The bell would ring, and I would start seeing little kids coming out of their classrooms.

Kids this age need a lot of reorientation in whatever they are doing. Once you give them direction, they follow very well. They need authority figures. There were plenty of those in the form of teachers and their aides. Each child was cuter than the other. My heart would swell with such cuteness overload.

I would look all around the school and dozens of little children forming lines to start going to the cafeteria. Some of them would be carrying lunch bags and others would be lining up in the cafeteria cue to buy their lunch.

My heart would race a little in the anticipation of seeing my daughter (and a few years later, my son.) Then there would be the moment when I would finally find my child in the crowd of kids.

As soon as my eyes met my daughter's, there would be a big smile on her face. I can still remember it being a shy smile. For her it would be a very big moment because her two lives would meet at this moment. Her school life and her home life.

Upon seeing her dad in front of her classmates, it was natural for her to feel a little shy and probably embarrassed too because something different was happening. Nobody else's dad was there but her dad was there. Sometimes she would be too shy to acknowledge me, and I would go over to her and hug her and other times she would break the line and come to me.

The school dining room was a long room with multiple tables and chairs. The kids had made small groups of friends and some of the friends would always sit with one another every day. The chairs were small and well suited for elementary school age children. I would look and feel like a giant from Gulliver's Travels sitting on those chairs.

In front of each child on the table were a variety of kids' foods like Goldfish crackers, peanut butter and jelly sandwiches, apple slices and flavored yogurt in kid-friendly packaging. There used to be two lunch ladies, one of them helping everyone with a big smile on her face and the other one with an annoyed frown and a wrinkled forehead.

Initially my daughter's little friends were shy and ate in silence, but they could not help staring at me with their big innocent eyes. My presence there was probably a big change in the monotony of their daily school lives.

Then one of them would muster up some courage to speak to me.

"Are you Zaina's dad?"

"Yes, I am! And what's your name?" I'd reply with a big smile.

"I'm Bella."

And then another girl would say her name and before you knew it all the girls around the table listening in to the conversation started telling me their names.

The lunchroom would become quite loud within a few moments and the frown-browed lunch lady would give out a loud holler for everyone to keep quiet while they finished their lunch. She'd have to do the same about every five minutes or so.

Lunch hour was not more than fifteen or twenty minutes. Soon as the bell rang, kids would start making lines again to get back to the classroom. I would kiss my daughter and hug her and say goodbye and go back to the front office to sign myself out.

On the drive back to work, I'd feel fulfilled as if I did not need anything more from that day. At the end of the workday when I would go back home and see my daughter again, we would smile with the memories of lunch that day.

For the next several months, I couldn't help but bring up memories from lunch. If she were to tell me a story about any of her friends, I would ask, "Is Leena the one who was wearing a big bow on her hair when I came to your school for lunch?"

I kept doing this a couple of times each year she was in elementary school. Then she graduated to middle school. She was excited and so was I. I went to middle school parent information night and the teachers did an excellent job of telling us what the kids would be studying and what their course materials would be.

The school building was really nice. The classrooms were comfortable, and each teacher had put on nice hangings on the walls pertaining to the subject that they were teaching. They also had us leave little notes in the desks for the kids that they would read in the morning.

They talked about the difference in the school philosophy between elementary and middle school where their emphasis was to give more independence and responsibility to the growing kids so that in a few years they were ready for high school and eventually for college.

They had also designed activities for the kids to equip them with the knowledge and skills of practical life such as giving them an assignment to do a load of laundry at home and to cook a basic meal even if it was to fry an egg for breakfast.

I was quite impressed by the thought that was put into designing such a comprehensive curriculum for the kids, until the end of the presentation when they asked us parents if we had any questions.

Never being shy to state my mind or ask questions when in a group, I swiftly raised my hand. The teacher diverted her attention to me and signaled with a nod for me to ask my question.

"I'm looking at my daughter's daily schedule and there are two time periods in the afternoon that show up as free time. One of them is probably lunch time and the other says study hall which I assume is when they are given time to study. Can I come to spend time with my daughter in either one of the two periods or can I come just during lunch time?" I inquired.

"Well parents are not allowed to have lunch with their kids during school hours, sorry," she responded.

For a moment I could not believe what she said.

"I'm sorry I don't understand. You mean I cannot have lunch with my daughter during school days anymore?" I asked with a puzzled look on my face.

"Yes, you heard that right. There are several other ways that you can decide to spend time with your child during school. You can consider volunteering for different activities which happen during school hours and also after-school activities. If you want to talk to your child's teachers, all you need to do is contact them and they will be happy to schedule a time to meet you and address any concerns or questions that you might have."

"Why do you have a policy like that? Is it at the school level or the district level?" I inquired.

"You will have to call our main line and ask to speak with someone in the Superintendent's office to know the answer. I assume it's for the safety of your own child sir. We try to restrict the number of non-student visitors in the school. Also middle school is a bit different than elementary school and here we try to make the kids more independent and start getting ready for the real world out there. When they are seniors in high school, they can be allowed to leave school premises for lunch and you can spend time with them if you wish," she explained.

I did not see any value in prolonging this conversation, so I just stayed quiet in return. But in my mind, I felt sad and discouraged. One of the things that I enjoyed the most as a parent was being taken away from me.

My mind drifted to the times when during the COVID pandemic, the hospitals were not allowing visitors with elderly patients to prevent the spread of infection, but the family members found it very hard not be at their parents' bedside and that too at a very critical and vulnerable time where they needed their company the most.

During the rest of the years that my daughter was in school, I never got a chance again to go and have lunch with her. I thought of participating in some other ways such as volunteering but it did not come easy to me.

Once I signed up to be a cashier at the pizza stand at a school event but that's all I ended up doing. I could not spend any time with my daughter.

Also most other parent volunteers were moms and as a single dad, I felt quite out of place. Some other dads were coaching after school activities such as sports or boy scouts, but I simply was not interested in those activities. I simply wanted to have lunch with my child which I couldn't.

. . .

As I walk past my daughter's bedroom a dozen times during the day, I can sense the emptiness and the silence that it now represents.

Sometimes I open the door and take a look inside just to make sure that all her things are in order. I look at the well-made bed with some of her stuffed toys laying on top looking cute but motionless.

I look at her desk and chair which has not been used in days. I look at her closet filled with clothes waiting to be worn again some day.

The whole room appears to share my longing for her to visit again as soon as she can and as frequently as her college commitments allow.

I think how in just a matter of another few years, my son will also be gone to college, and I will enter a new phase of my life.

Being an eternal optimist, I look forward to the next "empty nester" phase of my life which will hopefully bring with a lot of free time that I can spend on myself pursuing various hobbies and activities such as travel, things that I could not previously do because of having to take care of the kids.

I'm sure I will be able to adapt to the new phase and make the most out of it but that doesn't take away from the fact that the previous phase will be gone. The phase when my kids were little, and life was all about taking care of them in every possible way.

As I look back at that phase of life, even though I put all that I had into rearing these kids, I still think about things that I could have done more.

Could I have played more tennis with my daughter? Could I have watched more cartoons with my son? Could I have spent less time on my phone? Could I have gone out with my friends less and spent more time at home reading with the kids?

But these are all the things that I could control. The middle school not letting me have lunch with my child was not in my control. It was a restriction that was imposed upon me by an institution that I was sending my kids to, and I had to abide by their rules and regulations.

Should I have gone to more school meetings and advocated for parent-child lunches during school hours? Should I have put together a group of like-minded parents and tried to arrange a meeting with the Superintendent? Was I the only parent who was wishing to have lunch with my child?

A school's goal should be to constantly find ways for the parents to be more involved in their school lives. Already there are a lot of concerns across the board that kids may be learning things in school that the parents wouldn't necessarily want them to.

Conservative parents worry about the "woke" ideology that the kids learn in schools in liberal districts. The opposite is also true when liberal parents find their kids start espousing conservative ideas and blame the schools and teachers for that.

You would think that if parents' involvement in school activities is increased, the gap could be bridged a little more effectively.

When I look at my kids and see them grow into the amazing young adults that they are now, I cannot thank their school enough. They provided them with all the tools to have successful, happy and good lives. They nurtured them into quality individuals.

Yes, they say that it takes a village to raise a child but the primary two entities in the entire village doing that are the parents and the teachers. Teachers can be given equal if not more credit than parents to shape up the personalities of the children.

But if I were to be given a survey about the overall job that the American Middle School did at training my child, I would have given a ten on a performance scale but I'm sorry to say that I will have to give a nine, simply because I still think that they should have let me have lunch with my child.

Essays by a Human

A Gift from Gloria to Rabia

The house that I live in is an old house. It was built in 1939. It is in one of the older neighborhoods in town.

Most people that live here are older in age and have been living here for decades. The couple who used to live here, who we bought the house from, became empty-nesters and then retired and the house was too much work for them, so they decided to move to a smaller place in another part of town.

When it was put up for sale, as soon as we looked at it with our realtor, we fell in love with the hundred-year-old trees in the backyard and the character of the entire house.

It was a nice break from the "cookie-cutter" American houses. Having a feeling of love at first sight, we placed an offer that was accepted, and we moved in right away.

It is sometimes nice to have neighbors who have kids that are the same age as yours. The kids have company and parents also have similar interests.

But we discovered after we moved in that most of our neighbors were older people that were our parents' age. I thought this was nice because it would mean more of a quiet and mature neighborhood without much partying by teenagers or chaos from little kids running around.

Our next-door neighbors stopped by to introduce themselves. John was a lawyer who had retired a few years ago and Gloria had a career in education. It was a second marriage for both of them.

Their children were my age who lived nearby and visited them often. They often hosted the grandkids on weekends and would set up their yard with games for them to play. They gave us their phone numbers to keep handy in case we needed anything and told us that they were always there for us but they also value privacy, both theirs and ours and would not "butt-in" too much into our business.

Our backyard was beautiful and huge. The trees were old, large and with abundant leaves resulting in the most beautiful shade. There were a lot of plants that were perennials and with flowers of different types and colors, added to the beauty of the garden.

The patio was small but cute and classy and I knew that this would be the place of countless friends and family get-togethers around bonfires.

This all was good until the time came to mow the lawn and attend to the upkeep of the plants. It took me about an hour to mow the lawn which was initially quite enjoyable. It felt as if I was making love to my land or grooming a body part.

The satisfaction that a woman draws from having cleaned the house and walking into a sparkly, tidy kitchen or living room; similar is the feeling of a man after he mows the yard, and I couldn't help but stare at the freshly cut grass in neat patterns.

However, I soon realized that it would require too much of my time to take care of the yard all by myself and I had to hire a landscaping company to mow my lawn and to keep the plants in decent shape.

As much as I liked my own backyard but no matter what I did, I could not make it look as nice as John and Gloria's. Gloria was retired and you could find her meticulously and passionately working in her backyard all the time.

It almost felt like if there was daylight and if she was awake, you could find her in her garden. It was no surprise that her flower beds, grass and trees looked like they belonged to the centerfold of a housekeeping magazine.

But every time I would look at her garden, I could not help but think that my garden, although pretty decent by my standards, was looking so mediocre and unkempt compared to hers. I knew I was being silly thinking that way.

Gloria was retired and had all the time in the world, plus gardening was her passion. This was not a matter of making comparisons. But my mind would not budge from the thought that as people drove by our street, they would marvel at the beauty of her garden and then my front yard would stick out like a sore thumb tarnishing the beauty of the neighborhood.

It was a nice beautiful sunny day. I came out for a walk in my backyard. I was looking at some of the plants and admiring their beauty, thanking my luck that they were very low maintenance plants, and I did not even have to water them. The rain every few days took care of it.

I turned around and saw Gloria walking towards me. She was carrying a small pail of water and some gardening tools.

"Your garden is looking nice," she remarked.

"Not nearly as nice as yours Gloria," I replied thinking that while she was being courteous, she must really be thinking how much work needs to be done in my garden.

"Well I spend a lot of time in my garden. If you put your time and your heart towards it, your garden could look better than mine." That was a nice way of her saying how she thought my garden sucked.

"I do so many other things and then I have to drive the kids around for their activities. That does not leave me too much time to spend in the garden." I made the usual excuse.

"See that flower bed in the corner? There are some weeds sticking out and if you pull them out, it will look so much better," she pointed out.

"I know I will try to get to it next weekend." I was feeling embarrassed that my garden had weeds. But on the other hand I told myself that there is no way that I'm spending my hours plucking weeds in the garden.

I had many other things to do and to be honest, the flower bed looked pretty nice to me. Maybe it was not up to her standards, but I was perfectly comfortable with how it looked.

"Also that brown spot in your front yard. That's probably because that part of the yard gets a lot of sun. Maybe you should water it more often. And also check with your landscaping company what kind of weed killer they are putting in your yard. Maybe it is too strong for your grass." She seemed not to run out of things to point out in my yard that in her opinion needed immediate attention.

"I know it's your garden but when I'm pruning my plants later today, I can clean up this flowerbed for you if you don't mind," she offered.

"Oh by all means Gloria. I don't know when I will get to it but if you have some extra time, please feel free to do whatever you want. There is a saying in Spanish, "Mi Casa, Su Casa" which means, my house is your house. So consider my yard as your yard and anything that you would like to do to improve it, I don't mind one single bit," I replied.

She never did.

. . .

The summer went by. My friends visited me almost every weekend and we loved sitting around a fire on my garden patio. I put a hammock under the shade of the big old trees, and it was very peaceful to spend a hot afternoon in the shade of the trees reading a book while sipping on an ice-cold beverage.

One day as I got up from the garden to go inside the house after the sun started going down, I saw Gloria approaching me in the shared driveway. She was holding a sizable book in her hands.

"You were saying the other day that you don't know too much about gardening. Well there is always somewhere to start with. Here, I have had this book since I started gardening a million years ago and it has helped me learn everything about gardening. I want you to have the book and learn from it just like I did. I'm sure you will love it." She handed over the book to me.

It was a large hardcover book of about five hundred illustrated glossy pages. It was called, *'The American Horticultural Society – Encyclopedia of Gardening.'* I love books and I have my own personal library and every time I get my hands on a book, I don't miss an opportunity to borrow it or steal it and add it to my library even if I plan never to read it.

But here she was giving me this book which, if I took from her, would imply that I had to start using it. It meant having to spend more time working in the garden, which I had absolutely no plans for.

"Thank you, Gloria, I really appreciate you sharing this book with me, but it must be very personal to you specially if you have had it for so long. This summer, I might not have much time to spend in the garden so I'm not sure how much I will end up using it," I said.

"It's ok you can have it; you can use it whenever you feel like it. I promise you that you will learn a lot from it," she replied.

I had to take the book. I thanked her again and brought it home. I browsed through some of the pages and then set it aside on the table.

A few days later when I was tidying up the room, I put it in a bottom shelf in the library that had space for a bigger, taller book and it sat there for the next few years.

. . .

One day I went to work and, in the patient waiting room, I saw Gloria sitting there alone waiting for her turn to be called in to be seen by the doctor. I knew that it was not a good sign for her to be a patient at the cancer center.

I knew she valued her privacy so I was reluctant to walk up to her but then decided that I should go and ask.

"Hi Gloria. Is everything okay? What are you doing here at the Cancer Center?" I asked.

"Oh I'm okay. I was diagnosed with colon cancer a few months ago and I had to have it surgically removed. The doctors are telling me that it's all taken care of, but I have to see the doctor and have scans every few months to make sure it doesn't come back. It is hard to go through surgery at my age, but I think I'm doing fine now," said Gloria.

"Well you know I work here so if I can be of any help, please let me know. I know the doctor who you are seeing, and he is a great guy and I'm sure he will take good care of you," I told her.

"Thank you," she simply said.

. . .

I didn't get to see John and Gloria a lot during the winter months. The freezing temperatures were by no means any incentive to venture outdoors. Our gardens would be covered by inches of snow anyways.

Gloria probably had some indoor plants that she tended to during the winters to remain engaged in her favorite hobby. During springtime when the snow melted and the leaves started sprouting from the plants, Gloria would make a reappearance in her garden.

I saw her walking on her driveway inspecting her plant beds.

"Hi Gloria, long time no see," I greeted her.

"Hi Farhan. Good to see you. When the snow melts, we get to say hi to each other. How have you been?" she replied.

"I'm doing great. Listen, it's been on my mind all winter to tell you that I still have your gardening book. I haven't been able to use it much and I have hired a company to manage my garden this year so I will not be using it much. It's a very expensive book and you have had it for such a long time. I wouldn't want it just sitting there collecting dust. Can I give it back to you?" I asked.

"You know, it's the kind of a book that if you keep it, I'm sure that some day you will find the use of it. Maybe if you keep it, it will serve as a reminder every now and then for you to consider it as your next hobby," she replied.

"I know but if that happens, I can always take it back from you?" I asked.

"Let's do this. You either keep it and use it yourself some day or maybe any of your kids might start taking interest in gardening. Maybe you can give it as a gift to someone who really enjoys gardening and will make use of it," she suggested.

I thought in my mind, 'Okay that's enough! I have offered it back to her and she is not taking it back. I'm just going to keep it and not bring it up again unless she asks for it herself.'

The book remained on the same shelf in the library, occasionally being moved to another shelf whenever I was tidying up my library and rearranging books.

. . .

I came home from work one day and parked my car in the garage. I walked to the mailbox to retrieve the mail and as I was walking back, Gloria's son Jack drove by in his truck.

Jack was about my age and was always smiling and cheerful. He often visited his parents, and his kids would play all day in their backyard. He waved at me and slowed down his truck to a stop.

"How's it going Jack? How's work?" I asked.

"Work is just fine. I'm just trying to visit my parents most days of the week after work now," said Jack.

"That's so nice of you. See, my parents live so far away that I cannot visit them frequently, but I call my mom every day on my way to work," I said.

"Well I'm not sure if you know or not but my mom is in the hospice. She has only a few more weeks left to live according to the doctors," he said.

"Oh my God! I didn't know that. I am so very sorry to hear that. I hope she is not in too much pain. I am hoping I can stop by to see her one of these days, if that's okay?" I asked.

"Sure I will ask my parents, but you know that they value their privacy a lot."

He drove away but left me with a very uneasy and confused feeling. I kept thinking to myself that my next-door neighbor was on her deathbed, and I did not even know about it.

What kind of a neighbor was I? Wasn't it supposed to be my responsibility to know if any of my neighbors was going through a difficult time?

Ever since I was a child, at home and at school it was taught that in order to be a good human being, helping others and being there for them at times of need takes more importance than anything else in life.

So ignorant was I, of the woes of my neighbor, that I was just learning about her being at the end of her life by a casual drive-through conversation with her son.

I came home and partially intentionally created a panic-like situation at home. I thought of it as an opportunity to teach kids how important it is to be there for our neighbors. I told them that Gloria was dying, and she only had a little time left and that we had to do everything to make her feel loved and cared.

We thought of preparing some food but then decided against it because we didn't know what her dietary restrictions would be at this physical state.

We thought of getting her flowers and visiting her but then I realized how her son had said that his parents really value their privacy.

Did he mean that they would not want visitors and by visiting her, I would be inconveniencing them?

Finally I decided to write a letter. I wrote down my thoughts and emotions and well wishes to her. I had my kids also add a paragraph each about how they felt. In the letter I left my cell number saying that if Gloria was in a condition that she was willing to take visitors, to let us know. I left the letter in their mailbox.

I did not hear back from either John or Jack.

A few days later I saw a number of cars gathered outside her house and learnt that these were all close family members who were visiting because she had breathed her last.

. . .

A few months ago I was talking to my friends on a WhatsApp video call. We were planning our next get-together. We talked about visiting some country in South America or Europe where we had not been to before.

Everyone was scrambling to find time on their busy schedules to take time off for a friends' reunion. I suggested that this time they visit me because Western New York becomes so beautiful in the summers.

They would also get to visit Toronto and Montreal since they were close to me and finally, they made a plan to visit me in Rochester.

A few days before their arrival, I got a call from Asad. Asad has been my friend since elementary school. Not only is he my friend but we were also neighbors as kids, family friends and since both our fathers were physicians, we had a very similar childhood.

"Is there a shopping area or a mall close to where you live?" he asked.

"Of course, yes, there is a nice mall only ten minutes from me. What do you need?" I asked.

"I want to buy a gift for Rabia. Right after I come back from our trip, it's our anniversary and I haven't bought a gift yet. Also if you have any nice gift ideas, let me know," he said.

My mind wandered to the time when we were in high school, and Asad had newly fallen in love with Rabia. Asad was a popular guy and Rabia became the envy of many girls.

Asad and I both had similar tastes in music and even today we tell each other how he introduced me to the music of Elvis, and I introduced him to Mehdi Hassan. One day Shania Twain's song "You're still the one" was playing and he was really enjoying it.

He turned to me and said, "Every word of this song is so true."

"It doesn't really do anything for me," I replied.

"How could it not?" He asked.

"Not everybody gets lucky in love like you did Asad. There are many people who either do not end up getting the person that they love or even if they do, they might fall out of love at some point," I elaborated.

Having been with Rabia for more than two decades now, he was probably still enjoying the song and looking for a gift to celebrate yet another anniversary.

My friends finally arrived at my place. It was after a long time that we had met. We were sitting in my living room where I have made one wall into a library. It is a large wall with close to a thousand books in the collection.

I thought that we would spend the day at home and have a nice dinner and the next morning I would take Asad to the mall to help him find a gift for Rabia.

As we were talking, I saw Asad browsing through the books in the library. His eyes stopped at one book. "This book looks interesting." He got up and pulled that book from the shelf.

I could not believe it when I saw that out of a thousand books, the one book that he picked up was The Encyclopedia of Gardening – the same book that Gloria had given me.

He excitedly started flipping through the pages and mumbling to himself, "Rabia will love this book. She is really into gardening."

"Well in that case we don't have to go to the mall anymore. That book right there would be the best gift for her. Maybe it has been sitting on that shelf all these years, waiting to find its appropriate owner," I said.

. . .

Was this a mere coincidence or should I take it as a spiritual experience?

Aristotle would say that gardening is a very common hobby, and it would have been very natural for Asad to choose a book out of others that aligned with his and Rabia's interests.

The book is large-sized and was fairly prominent amongst other books and it was quite natural for him to be drawn to this book and that is why he picked it out from the entire library.

It was a coincidence that it was the same book that Gloria had given to me to eventually gift it to someone.

Plato would say that something else is going on. In some other world, such as his world of otherworldly Forms, maybe this was intended to be a gift from Gloria to Rabia.

I had tried my best to return the book to Gloria thinking that I had no use for it, but Gloria had insisted that I keep the book and maybe someday give it to someone who would actually like it and make good use of it.

At that time I had no idea who I would give it to. I had even thought that if I ran out of space, I would donate the book to a public library but maybe the book came into my house with its own destiny.

It was meant to be given by Gloria to Rabia in the first place; and for it to come to my library and for Asad to visit me, after all these years, were merely events that were vehicles for the delivery of this gift from one woman to the other who had never met each other but in some spiritual realm, were connected to each other through their common passion of gardening.

. . .

We often hear from people about certain spiritual experiences that they go through. I personally have never had one. I'm always looking for something like that to happen to me. It just doesn't happen. Or maybe I don't look correctly. Maybe this story was as close to being a "spiritual" experience as possible.

You must be thinking what I mean by having a spiritual experience. Let me try to explain.

If you pick up any book on western philosophy, the central figure is Socrates. The chapters are usually divided into pre-Socratic philosophers and the ones that came after him. The trio of Socrates followed by Plato and Aristotle hold the most central role in all of western philosophy.

Socrates himself did not write anything, but Plato and Aristotle wrote prolifically, and their teachings are considered the basis of all or most knowledge that we still have today.

Their concepts were taken and rehashed in a million ways by subsequent philosophers resulting in the knowledge that humankind has today.

During the sixteenth century Renaissance period, the famous artist Raphael was commissioned to draw some paintings called frescos for the Pope's palace. One of the paintings he made was called "The School of Athens."

In this painting he painted multiple philosophers representing all the "big shots" of philosophy known until that time.

At the center of the painting are Plato and Aristotle symbolizing their central role in all philosophical thought. Plato is seen as an older man while Aristotle is young, reminding us how the latter was the former's student. Aristotle learned from Plato all his life but towards the end rejected some of his theories and came up with his own philosophy.

Both of them are seen holding their own authored books in their hands which are still some of the most widely read texts around the world.

Now if you look closer, Plato is pointing towards the sky, but Aristotle has his hand pointed towards the earth almost in a manner as if to rebuke Plato.

Just by the gesture of the hands, Raphael has managed to show the most basic difference in the core concepts of the philosophies of both the great thinkers.

The reason Plato is pointing towards the sky is because Plato tells us that this world that we live in, is not the real world. This is just a temporary illusion. There is a real world out there called the world of Forms.

What we see here is only a reflection, just like a shadow that a caveman would see on the wall of a cave without being able to see the original object that he is seeing the shadow of.

The world is much more than what we can see with our eyes or can feel with our senses. There is another so-called spiritual or metaphysical world out there that is not visible to our eyes.

Aristotle on the other hand, is pointing towards this world and suggesting that what we see, and experience is simply what it is. He relies on his senses and starts categorizing worldly things in an orderly manner.

His work became the basis and the starting point of all the sciences that we have today. He gave us the most basic, initial concepts of the fields of ethics, politics and economics.

One can easily say that his work is the foundation of all the different academic subjects that we have today.

Oversimplifying something runs the risk of misunderstanding a concept but it still helps with beginning to comprehend an issue at hand.

In our day-to-day world, I like to apply Raphael's depiction of Plato and Aristotle in a broad way. To me, whenever somebody tells me that they had an "other worldly" or so-called spiritual or metaphysical experience, I feel that they are being Platonic.

When people talk of seeing spirits or ghosts, djinns or angels, they are talking about beings that are not visible to the eye, but they say that they exist. There are psychics who claim to read others' minds and predict the future.

Sometimes we have premonitions or get a feeling about something without any factual evidence, and we call it the sixth sense. There is no proof of these things but still these are widely believed by humans. Nobody has seen the soul, but everybody says that it exists.

But if you were to ask Aristotle, he would argue that we should work with what we have at hand in this world. We should rely on our senses to see and feel the material things that surround us and go deeper into their study. This is what all the scientists and engineers and other professionals are doing every day of their lives.

Fatima

"Today is a special day, Emily. Maybe one of the most important days of your life." I tried to conclude the clinical encounter. After giving her scientifically derived percentages of prognosis of her breast cancer and answering all her carefully jotted-down questions, I tried to end with a customary parting comment.

"It's been almost a year since you found this lump in your armpit and look at how it changed your entire life. Everything changed. It changed how you think; what you do; how you look at life now. How you have beaten this cancer but are still scared. How you are physically weaker but so much mentally stronger now. You went through a year of surgeries, chemotherapy and radiation and finally today is your last treatment," I added.

"I want you to be happy today. Go please celebrate with your friends and family. But that is the easy part. I'm going to ask you to do something that will not come that easy unfortunately. I want you to forget about your cancer. The cancer can indeed come back but you have done everything to reduce your chances of recurrence. Now it is going to play with your mind. Even more so than before.

Now you will have to live a life where you will often not be able to shake off this unwelcome thought of the cancer's ability to come back any time. There will be moments when you will realize that the crook has invaded your mental space and is trying to break through all the defense mechanisms that you have built. At that moment I want you to identify this thought and then isolate it, roll it up into a ball and throw it right out of the window and move on with your happiness. I know, easier said than done, but that is a fight you will have to fight for the rest of your life," I explained.

"Thanks for everything you have done for me," replied Emily. "But please tell me what else can I do so that this cancer doesn't ever come back? Should I go on a specific diet?"

This is a very common question that almost every cancer survivor asks. With my years of experience in clinical medicine, I had a well-rehearsed answer and had taught many medical students "how to counsel a cancer survivor."

Just like everything in medicine, such as defined algorithms of clinical management, the prognostic percentages in clinical trials, the lists of side effects and drug interactions, doctors are also trained at giving research-based lifestyle recommendations to cancer survivors.

"Well there is no specific diet that you have to go on. You just try to eat healthy, exercise as much as you can, push yourself to the limit and stay away from the three toxins that majority of the humans are destroying their own bodies with: tobacco, alcohol and food. On top of that, my team and I will see you once a year and periodically order blood work and scans to make sure you are cancer-free. That's it!" I outlined her surveillance plan.

At this point I felt that I had covered everything and that they should not have been left with any more questions to ask.

"And don't forget prayer, Doctor." Her husband interjected as Emily reached out for his hand as a tear rolled down her cheek.

"Yes of course!" I responded as my mind wandered to the NCCN guidelines that oncologists follow all over the world (put forth by the National Comprehensive Cancer Network, an organization composed of some of the most intelligent minds in the world currently trying to beat cancer.) I could not recall "Prayer" as part of a surveillance plan for any type of cancer.

I have prayed with my patients before. Being an immigrant and also born and raised into a different religion compared to that of most of my patients, it took me years to become somewhat comfortable engaging into a discourse with my patients about religion and spirituality.

"Who do you pray to? How will you pray?" I asked.

"We are Roman Catholic. We are actually flying to Portugal. Sort of a pilgrimage," he replied.

I scoured my brain for any information related to the significance of Portugal in Christianity but couldn't come up with anything owing to the paucity of knowledge about the history of Catholicism.

I knew that Muslims go to Mecca and Jews go to Jerusalem for pilgrimage but other than the Vatican, I did not know of any other places that Christians go to for a major pilgrimage.

"What's in Portugal?" I inquired.

"There is this little town just north of Lisbon. It's called Fatima," he said.

My confusion doubled. Here I was, born and raised a Muslim, talking to some very devout Christians hearing a name from them that was already all too familiar to me. There couldn't be any other name more Muslim than Fatima. The daughter of the Prophet Muhammad (PBUH). The daughter of Khadija. The wife of Imam Ali. The mother of Imam Hassan and Imam Hussain. Grandmother to the Shiite Imams.

There is no other woman more central to the family of the Prophet Muhammad (PBUH) than Fatima. Not only a person of reverence for any Muslim but also as endearing as a daughter, wife or a mother.

Fatima is deeply entwined into early Islamic history and revered by all Muslims but specifically Shiites who consider her the mother of all the Imams to a point that in some parts of the Shia world, her birthday is celebrated as "Mother's Day."

"That's very interesting. Fatima is a very sacred name in Islam. What connection does Catholicism have with Fatima? Prophet Muhammad's (PBUH) daughter?" I asked.

"You know what? I don't know but I thought about that too. Next time I'm there, I will find out," he responded.

"Yes, I would love to know. Tell me what you find out when I see you for your next visit. Enjoy your travels. And your prayers," I said.

In this day of widely disseminated information, I did not need to or have the patience for waiting another six months for them to come back and give me the back story. I just opened another browser on my computer and typed in "Fatima" and all the information came up.

This reminded me of my grandfather who used to get frustrated when he could not find the answer to a historical question that would pop up in the middle of conversation.

He would try to look it up in one of the volumes of his Encyclopedia Britannica and often could not find the answer. He did not live to experience the magic and miracle of the phenomenon called "internet."

As I browsed through several different websites, I came to find out that this is actually a love story!

This is a tale from the eighth century. In the year 711CE the Iberian Peninsula that includes Spain and Portugal was conquered by Muslim invaders who came across the strait of Gibraltar.

One famous Arab conqueror was Tariq Bin Ziyad who famously had all his ships burnt after his army crossed so that they did not have retreat as an option.

Over the next few centuries there were ongoing battles between Christians and Muslims until eventually the land was recaptured by Christians.

During one of these battles, a Christian Knight by the name of Don Goncalo Hermingues captured the daughter of a Muslim Prince whose name was Fatima. They both fell in love, and she converted to Christianity. Her name was changed to Oureana after which the village of Ourem was named.

Tragically, only a few months after getting married, Fatima died, and Don Goncalo was heartbroken. He devoted the rest of his life to prayer and moved to the nearby mountains. He buried Fatima in the mountains and this town started being called Fatima, a tribute to her Muslim name.

More than a thousand years later, in 1917, three children from the village started saying that they were seeing the vision of Mary dressed in a white dress and shining with a bright light. The word got around and people started believing them. They could even predict when the apparitions of Mary would happen.

This led to an event when some 30,000 local people congregated based on a prophecy, on a specific date and reported the Sun to emit specific ways of lights called The Miracle of the Sun.

They built a temple at this site and called it "Our Lady of Fatima." The Roman Catholic Church later legitimized the account of the local people and designated the story "worthy of belief" resulting in about 6 to 8 million annual pilgrims to the shrine today.

I found this story to be such a fascinating link between the two matriarchal figures of both the major religions of the contemporary world.

As beautiful as I thought this tale was, I also wondered that as people will read this story, how they think about it will depict whether their hearts are filled more with love or hate.

Some Muslims will take this story not worthy of retelling because they would condemn the Moorish princess Fatima for apostasy.

Some Christians would use this story as a victory of sorts over Islam for a Muslim woman to have converted to Christianity.

But those Christians and Muslims who will have love in their heart, which I hope will be most of them, will take this story and retell it as a beautiful bridge between the two Abrahamic monotheistic faiths.

When Emily and her husband return for their next clinic visit, I will be ready to tell them what I read, and I will also be looking forward to hearing what stories they have to tell.

My Father wanted to be a Crow, I want to be an Ant

"In each human heart are a tiger, a pig, an ass and a nightingale. Diversity of character is due to their unequal activity." Ambrose Bierce (1842-1914)

This must have happened when I was hardly twelve years old. It was a usual Sunday late morning. We were sitting on the back porch of our house.

Over the course of your life, you end up living in different places, starting from your childhood home to dorm rooms to apartments and then on to your own house when you leave your parents' home. But the way that the childhood home resides into memory is different.

This is the home that often comes in your dreams. Our backyard was beautiful. It was neither too small nor too big. The best part was that in the winters, it got a lot of sunshine, and it was the most ideal place to be during the winter mornings and afternoons to soak up the warmth from the rays of the Sun.

My father was sitting at the edge of a bench, feet dangling and his home slippers on the floor right next to him. We were used to seeing him on the move at all times. During weekdays, he would leave home early and come back late at night. Even on weekends, he often had to leave for a few hours to work.

Seeing him sitting idly at the back porch was a relatively unusual sight. He must have been in his late forties, the same age as I am now. He was not a man of many words but that afternoon he said something that stuck to my mind. This was not a conversation. I don't know why he said it.

But it is one of those things that imprints on your mind and becomes part of your psyche. Looking into the sky, without any context, he said, "I wish I was a crow."

This is all I remember. There was no incident, no event. No conversation or monologue before or after. Just that one sentence and that's it.

For the rest of my life, from time to time, this phrase comes to my mind and makes me think about it. He lost his cognition multiple years before his death so when I grew up, I never got a chance to ask him why he said that.

There is also a pretty good chance that even if he was alive and well and if I had asked him, he might have said that he doesn't even remember when and why he said that. It may have been a very insignificant utterance for him but for some reason I could not shake it off of my head.

I now have my own interpretations of why he said it. Maybe he was too overworked, and this was his way of saying that if he was a bird, he would have been free from the duties a man has in this world.

The duties to get up in the morning, to work, to put food on the table. To follow rules, to make sense of world events, fulfill obligations and maintain relationships. Protect oneself and one's family from harm and danger.

Maybe he just wanted to be a free soul who had no deadlines to meet and no calendar to follow. He had achieved worldly success and had a good job. He was earning well and had a good reputation in his community. He had healthy children and had everything that a human can wish for.

But perhaps he was having a moment of questioning the reason for this existence. Maybe he was being lazy and just wanted to be on vacation. Maybe he wanted to win the lottery and retire on an island somewhere not having to work another day in his life.

That is all very understandable. We all have moments like that every once in a while, when we get overwhelmed with our current lives and schedules, worries and obligations and we wish for freedom from worldly entanglements.

But it still does not explain why he chose to be a crow. He could have wished to be any other animal or bird. He could have wished to be a butterfly, or a goat or a cat for that matter.

What was so special about being a crow? Did he just see a crow fly by? Or hear one caw? A crow cannot be considered one of the most beautiful or valuable birds out of the hundreds of thousands of species that are out there. It's actually one of the ugliest birds. There is nothing attractive about it. The sound that it makes is so annoying and jarring. It's a nuisance.

Fine. There might be some benefit to crows such as eating worms and pests that destroy crops. But still for farmers around the world, the crows remain largely a nuisance. That is why in many fields you have to erect a scarecrow. You don't have to erect a scare sparrow or a scare parrot or a scare falcon, but scarecrows are everywhere.

In most places where the department of energy conservation regulates the limits of how many birds one can hunt per day, depending on how much they have to conserve their population, there is no limit on how many crows a hunter can kill. This speaks to the uselessness of this bird.

In horror movies, if they have to show an abandoned and spooky place, they usually show it infested with crows and ravens. When they show rotten dead bodies in movie scenes, they are shown being eaten by vultures and crows. They are the ultimate scavengers and will eat from heaps of garbage and filth.

I know I'm being too harsh on crows. They may not be all that bad and every form of life in this world should be considered beautiful and with a purpose.

But how do I reconcile the properties of a crow with what my father uttered that idle morning? He is not there for me to ask him anymore so how do I make sense of this memory that has been ingrained in my mind.

Should I just think that he meant nothing by it? Should I think that he wanted to be an insignificant form of existence?

Maybe he thought that there is a certain feeling of freedom associated with being a crow. Maybe you do not have to strive to be your best at all times. Maybe he did not want to have the pressure of looking good or sounding good.

Maybe he wanted to be a being from whom nobody has any expectations. Maybe he did not care about the ugliness and uselessness of the crow, and he still loved crows. Maybe that is the exact reason why he loved crows more than other supposedly more "worthy" birds and animals.

. . .

We live in a vast universe. There are many purported explanations of this existence in the form of philosophies, religions and scientific postulates. Yet there is none.

In this world, humans have thought of themselves as the center of the universe. For a long time, it was thought that the Sun and the stars rotate around the Earth. The meaning of existence was thought to revolve around the human being.

In the seventeenth century, when originally Copernicus and later Galileo showed with the advent of the telescope that it was actually the Earth that revolved around the Sun and later with advancing technology, we came to find out that the Sun is just one of billions of stars in this vast universe, the existence of humans seems so insignificant and trivial.

The Earth as it was seen for the first time by astronauts from a distance, was called the "Pale Blue Dot," appearing just as a dust speck that you see in the rays of sunshine after brooming the living room. Such was the opposition to these views that Galileo was persecuted and placed on house arrest.

Rene Descartes, who is considered one of the most profound thinkers in western philosophy from the times of the French Enlightenment, withdrew his book from publication, worried about being persecuted for his views after he saw what was done to Galileo.

Such is the level of self-importance in humans' minds that we consider ourselves a superior species compared to all other forms of existence in the world.

We eat other animals, incarcerate them, use their furs and skins to make clothes and furniture. We torture them and breed them, keeping them in horrible conditions for human consumption. We claim that we have a higher intellect than all other animals.

How did we reach this conclusion? The obvious answer is that we can do things that other animals cannot. We can speak. We can talk. We study science, arts and history. We wear clothes. We get embarrassed. We tell stories. We cook our meals. We count days and months and years. We make ourselves cozy homes to live in.

We travel from one place to another using other animals or machines. We build buildings and we come up with ways to treat others who are ill, and we try to live longer. We try to explore space. We make weapons to kill each other in large numbers. We try to dominate the world.

But who has come up with the definition of intelligence? We ourselves. If we were to conduct a scientific study to test the level of our intelligence as a species, who would our control arm be? A goat? Or fish? Maybe an owl?

Yes, we do seem to ourselves as more intelligent than these control arm animals but that is not a very high standard to achieve. In the big scheme of things, what purpose have we achieved by doing all these things that other animals cannot do?

We are the only species that has to pay for where we live. We have to pay for our food and clothes. We are the only ones who become depressed and cry and be miserable. We are the only ones who kill each other in mass numbers. We are the only ones who seek world domination. We are the only ones who give each other hate in the form of racism.

Does that make us more or less intelligent compared to other animals? Maybe if you change the definition of intelligence from measuring the so-called "intelligence quotients" to measuring happiness and freedom from the intricacies of the human mind, we might conclude that we are less intelligent than most other animals on the planet. Maybe the human brain is not a blessing but rather a curse. A curse that has been given in such a form that we value it as the most precious part of human existence, but it is actually the same mind that is leading to such misery.

I once had a question in my mind as to which animals have the highest level of intelligence. I looked it up and of course humans have done studies to see which animals have the highest level of intelligence. Monkeys, chimpanzees, dolphins, elephants, pigs, owls. All these animals are considered to have a level of intelligence that is above others.

But these studies are done by giving these animals tasks and seeing how intelligently they perform these tasks such as navigation if they are lost or their ability to solve very simple problems.

I think that if we look at their behavior in a slightly different way, we might reach a different conclusion as to the level of intelligence of animals.

If we measure their intelligence in regard to how they deal with the most dangerous animal in the world, that is, the human, we may reach different answers. Humans have been a threat to almost every other form of life and existence in this world.

To achieve human comfort and longevity, most other forms of life, whether animals or plants, have been annihilated and destroyed and we continue to do so without any remorse.

To propagate human existence, we destroy forests and trees, we litter natural bodies of water, we kill animals and insects relentlessly. So, to me, the most intelligent animal would be the one that has learnt how best to tackle the most dangerous animal in the world also known as man.

By that standard, it appears that the dog and the cat are perhaps the most intelligent animals in the world. While other animals are out in the wild or being eaten by humans around the world, in a majority of the parts of the world, dogs and cats are living luxurious lives as pets in human households.

They are being fed delicious food, taken to the vets, their birthdays are celebrated, and their emotions are catered to. They live in warmed up houses and sleep in cozy beds. All this they have achieved by somehow over the centuries, convincing the human that they are great species to be kept at home as pets. How intelligent.

Applying the same standard to other animals, one can also conclude which animals are the dumbest. I wouldn't hesitate to put the chicken at the top of the list. Chicken is probably the most eaten animal by humans around the world. Neck to neck with the chicken would be the pig.

Not too far distant from these would be the cows and sheep. For some reason, their meat has blended best with human taste buds and unfortunately, they are killed and eaten more than any other animals. Such is their misery that humans don't let them get extinct, but we have come up with ways to breed them incessantly, keep them in horrific conditions and rather than allowing them to become extinct, we keep increasing their numbers to satisfy human consumption.

I would propose that we do not consider animals as less intelligent than humans. In many ways they can be considered more intelligent than us. That will give us an opportunity to think of them as equal living beings on this planet.

We can then have more empathy and love for all kinds of animals. That way we can also try to learn from each animal. We may not strive to be like one particular species of animals, but we can pick and choose different qualities from different animals and try to be like them in one way or another.

. . .

Cliched thoughts are considered to have a lack of originality. It is considered unattractive to not have genuineness of character and thought. One such cliche is to make new year's resolutions.

Mark Twain wrote, 'New Year's is a harmless annual institution, of no particular use to anybody save as a scapegoat for promiscuous drunks, and friendly calls, and humbug resolutions.'

It is commonly thought that people make new year's resolutions and try to follow them for the first few weeks of January and then forget about them and life moves forward in the unmotivated, unorganized way as usual. It is well known to try to avoid going to the gym in January because of crowds produced by such new year resolution enthusiasts.

But this is one of those cliche things that I still like to do. I love to make new year's resolutions. It is a great way to energize your mind and soul and to set up goals and targets.

If you end up achieving what you aimed and worked for, it brings a lot of joy and sense of accomplishment. If you don't achieve, it can serve as a good way to self-reflect on one's failures and to get oneself motivated to learn from mistakes and try to set up new goals in a more achievable way.

I was going through my journals and came across my new year's resolutions from the last several years.

Typically I divide them in various categories such as health goals or other goals pertaining to academic activities, relationships or other tasks such as learning to play musical instruments etc.

I noticed that although a few years ago, I had been successful in achieving a lot of my self-appointed goals, but in the last couple of years, my growth curves began stalling.

This gave me enough to think about where I was going wrong and what I could do to improve myself. I looked around to see who I could turn to who had shown levels of achievement that I could get inspiration from and try to be like them.

This is when, spontaneously the thought came to my mind that I wanted to be like an ant. I looked at the goals that I had ever failed to achieve.

Sometimes a goal is too vague, and it has to be made into a more tangible or achievable goal, but my goals were specific enough. Learn to play six songs on the piano this year. Run twenty miles a week. Read for an hour every morning. So I did not seem to have a problem with the specificity of the goals.

Other times the goals could be too overambitious. You may not be exercising at all and then make a new year's resolution to participate in an Ironman triathlon. A goal too unrealistic to achieve. I did not have that problem either. All my goals were attainable within a reasonable amount of time.

Was I lacking discipline to work on my goals? I did not think so either because I managed my time quite well. Then where was I going wrong? Why had my growth plateaued? After much thought,

I found my answer. I was giving in too much to the negative thoughts inside my own head.

Every man's capability of success in everything he does is directly proportional to his ability to suppress the negative voice that emanates from his own mind.

Every morning when you think about exercising, it is the negative in your own head that tells you that you are too tired.

If you are trying to call someone who you have not called in a few years, the only thing that stops you from doing so is your own voice in the head that says it would be awkward to call now, she has not called me so why should I call? What are we going to talk about when I call? Maybe they would not like it that I called.

And in the end, you do not make that call but if you suppress the negative thought in your own head and finally make the call, you feel so good about it. You are not only feeling good about rekindling that relationship but also feeling good about your own ability to overcome your negative self.

This way, you get rid of stagnation from your life. You move forward in your goals and desires and relationships. You achieve. You defeat negativity and procrastination. That brings happiness and fulfillment.

What other animal would be better to learn this from more than an ant. Look at the ant. It lives its life like it is on a mission. Always looks so determined and clear in its head. Look at its pace, its harmony and cooperation with other ants in its colony.

It works hard. If you put a rock in front of it, it will feel it a number of times, analyze it and then learn to walk around it and not let it come in the way of achieving its task. It will not break the workflow. It will not fight with another ant. It will not appear to be concerned whether it is doing more or less than other ants. Its focus seems to be on itself and its own improvement and achieving its own goals.

It will do its part in building an ant-nest. It will carry a speck of earth, as much as it has the capability to do so and bring it to the nest. It will carry a crumble of food half its own size, bring it to others to share and be happy without wanting to consume it all on its own or to hoard it for itself and deny it to other fellow ants.

You will never see it go out of line and try to break the discipline of the community. Its comparison is not with the other ants, but it is trying to be better than its own past self. It keeps its head down and is concerned only with the fulfillment of its own duties. It does not let its own negative self pull back on its desires and tasks at hand.

. . .

In a way, life is all about the pursuit of happiness. It is a good practice to train your mind to learn how to be happy from other people around us. The person does not necessarily need to be someone more educated than you or learned in some way. What you learn does not necessarily have to be in the form of a piece of knowledge or wisdom.

It could just be learning a way to do something or finding a new way to think about something. It could be the office janitor who is starting his night shift while you are finishing your work and heading home from whom you can learn how to always have a smile on your face and make time for small genuine talk in the middle of a busy day. It could be the distant aunt who you meet at the family gathering who takes pride in being on her feet all day and never wants to sit down.

It could be the neighbor's twelve-year-old daughter who celebrates her cat's birthday with such vigor and pomp. It could be the friend who you meet after such a long time who speaks only of positivity and makes a conscious effort not to let negative emotions bog him down.

Many philosophers have tried to come up with ways for humans to be happy. Aristotle, "The Philosopher," called this Eudemonia. He first defined the property that humans have that other animals don't, which is the ability to engage in a rational thought process.

He said that whatever task that humans are assigned to, if it is done in the best of ways, will bring happiness to us. For example if you are encountered with the task of baking a cake, it is neither too sweet nor too tasteless. It should have a color that is most pleasing to the eye. The size of it should be perfect for the intended number of people that will eat the cake. It should neither be too small so that some people go hungry nor too big so that half of the cake is wasted.

This method can be applied to anything that humans do using their rational thought process and intellect. He also called it "practical wisdom" suggesting that just being wise about doing something is not enough to achieve happiness. You have to put practicality to it. Knowledge is known to be power, but it is impotent unless if put into action.

Thereby, it is actually the execution of knowledge that is power. Knowledge without practicality and being put into action is nothing but stress and failure. Procrastination can lead to discontent and self-deprecation.

I would say that we should take it one step further and not just stop at learning from fellow human beings.

We should include animals in this endeavor. We can look around and observe the ways of different animals around us. We should see what they do better than humans. We could learn to be faithful from dogs. We could learn how to be selfish about our own comfort from cats.

We could learn to be industrious from ants. We could learn how to sing well from sparrows and nightingales. We could learn how to dance from butterflies.

Classic literature has numerous examples of animals as the main characters. Franz Kafka's protagonist becomes an insect in '*Metamorphosis*'. Charlotte is a spider that saves Wilbur the pig from slaughter in E. B. White's Charlotte's Web.

Considered as probably one of the best novels of the last century is '*Animal Farm*' where George Orwell describes the politics of a society through a whole slew of animal characters.

What did my father want to learn from being a crow, I still don't know. But I do know that this year I will strive to become more like an ant.

Maybe he was one of those people who derive satisfaction from doing nothing, floating through life like a plastic bag in the wind. Maybe I'm one of those people who love their checklists and daily goals which I would like to pursue day in and out with my head down, oblivious of my surroundings.

What animal would you like to be like?

Hell Hath no Fury Like a Woman Scorned

Some lines that you read or hear get stuck in memory without any good reason. From years of reading Sidney Sheldon books, the phrase "Hell hath no fury like a woman scorned" has been etched into my memory.

The idiom is sometimes attributed to Shakespeare but upon further digging I found out that this is a line from a seventeenth-century play called *"The Mourning Bride"* by William Congreve. The preceding line makes it complete:

Heaven has no rage like love to hatred turned, nor hell a fury like a woman scorned."

Recently I stumbled upon two incidents in religious history that reminded me of this phrase which I would like to share with you.

Ever since humans have inhabited this planet, for who knows how long, up until about two thousand years ago, most people in the world believed in many gods such as the Greco-Roman or Hindu polytheism.

However today, according to the Pew Research Center, about half of the world's population believes in one God. About 2.2 billion Christians and 1.6 billion Muslims believe in the one God of Abraham.

In the days of polytheism, it was common for humans to be considered as gods or demigods such as the Egyptian pharaohs or the Roman Emperors.

In today's world, only one human by the name of Jesus of Nazareth is considered God by billions of Christians around the world. Prophet Muhammad (PBUH) on the other hand, is not considered to be God by Muslims but carries the highest level of veneration any human can possibly have.

This is to the extent that even a slight mockery in any way will lead to violent protests around the world.

Recently I read the biographies of both Jesus and Prophet Muhammad (PBUH). Their stories are very well known to Christians and Muslims respectively, but I was able to curate two stories from their lives that represent atrocious acts of revenge and hatred, unified in their significance by virtue of the fact that they were committed by women.

If you are a Christian reading this essay, you are likely to know the story of Herodias but not that of Hind. If you are a Muslim, vice versa.

HERODIAS ANTIPAS

When is this story from?

Circa 29 CE

Who was she?

Herodias was the wife of King Herod Antipas – the ruler of Galilee in the early first century, during the life of Jesus.

Characters in this story:

–***John the Baptist:*** (Also known as Prophet Yahya by the Muslims) is a central figure in Christian history. He was a famous and influential Jewish preacher in the first century who lived in the area of and baptized people in the Jordan River. He had anticipated the arrival of the Messiah – the Savior of the Jewish people.

-Herod Antipas: Ruler of Galilee in the times of Jesus Christ. He was the son of King Herod the Great who had originally ordered the killing of all newborn boys in Bethlehem when the Magi priests predicted that the Messiah of the Jews would be born there.

-Salom: Herodias' teenage daughter from her previous marriage; Herod's stepdaughter.

What was Herodias' beef with John the Baptist:

John the Baptist publicly and vociferously condemned King Herod Antipas because he divorced his own wife and married his brother's wife Herodias. This was considered a blatantly sinful act by the Jewish people. Herod had John captured and thrown into prison at the mountaintop fortress at Machaerus. However, he decided not to have him killed, for fear of public retaliation. Herodias tried to persuade Herod to kill John, but he did not think it was a good idea.

What happened?

One day, King Herod Antipas invited the nobles of town to his fortress in order to celebrate his birthday. After dinner, he surprised his guests by asking Salom to present a dance. She performed so beautifully that everybody in attendance was in awe. King Herod, holding his head high with pride, proclaimed, "Ask me for anything you want, and I will give it to you!"

Salom was young and naïve and like most young girls, goes straight to her mother and puts the decision in her hands, "What should I ask for?" At this time, Herodias could have asked for anything, knowing that King Herod had given his word in front of all the nobles of the city and would not be able to let her down.

She decided to quench the thirst of revenge and sent Salom back to King Herod. "I want the head of John the Baptist." Everybody in attendance gasped with horror. The King was reluctant to kill John for political and religious reasons but had no choice but to fulfill his promise and ordered his men to behead John. John was forced to his knees and an executioner severed his head with his sword and presented it to Herodias and Salom on a silver platter. Thus, one of the noblest men in Jewish and Christian history fell prey to the scorn and fury of a slighted woman.

HIND BINT UTBA

When is this story from?

Circa 625 CE

Who was she?

Hind was a woman of importance in the Quraysh tribe to which Prophet Muhammad (Peace be upon him PBUH) belonged. She was the wife of Muhammad's uncle Abu Sufyan who held a high position and was the leader of the Meccans that fought against early Muslims. She was also the mother of Muawiya who was initially given the coveted post of Governor of Syria and after Ali's death, became the ruler of the Muslim Ummayad rule. She was also the grandmother of Yazid who was the central figure in the tragedy of martyrdom of Muhammad's grandson Hussain.

Characters in this story:

-Hamza: He was Muhammad's uncle and a ferocious warrior. Nobody dared come close to him on the battleground because of his masterful combat skills.

-Wahshi Ibn Harb: He was an Ethiopian slave who initially fought against but eventually embraced Islam.

What was Hind's beef with Hamza?

Hind was seething in the fire of revenge because Hamza had killed her father and brother in the Battle of Badr.

What happened?

At the Battle of Uhd, Hind commissioned Wahshi to find Hamza at the battleground and kill him. "Come on, black man! Satisfy your vengeance and ours!" For Wahshi, it was not easy to get close to Hamza because this would be like an act of suicide, but he was promised to be freed if he accomplished this task. Freedom's worth was more to him than his life, so he summoned courage and found Hamza on the battleground.

He threw his spear at him that went through the abdomen of an unsuspecting Hamza, exiting between his legs and he fell to the ground. Wahshi knew that he got Hamza and returned to Hind to inform her of the good news. Hind was still not satisfied and wanted to see it with her own eyes.

She went to the battleground after the battle was over. Walking over freshly killed and mutilated bodies, she went around trying to find Hamza's body. She uttered a shrieking chant when she found the body:

"You, O Wahshi, have assuaged the burning in my breast. I shall thank Wahshi as long as I live until my bones rot in the grave."

She, along with some other women, disfigured the corpses and made necklaces and beads out of cut-off noses and ears. She dug her dagger into Hamza's body and gouged out the liver and chewed on it, blood dripping over her mouth and chin onto her neck and chest.

Although later after Mecca was conquered by Muhammad, she accepted Islam and had a useful role in the Battle of Yarmouk, her son Muawiya was called the "Son of the Liver Eater" behind his back even when he was the most important man in the Muslim world, as the ruler of the Muslim dynasty in the seventh century.

Just saying:

Out of all the things that God has made for man in this world, the most beautiful indeed, is a woman. Nothing gives more happiness and joy to a man than a woman, be it in the form of a mother, a sister, a daughter, a wife, or a lover. But make no mistake. Be careful so as not to spite a woman, because:

Hell hath no fury like a woman scorned.

(This essay was written on the seventh day of the month of June, two thousand and twenty-three years since the time when Jesus was a child and in three decades would make his final journey from Capernaum to Jerusalem. This is also written on the eighteenth day of the month of Dhul Qidah, one thousand four hundred and forty-four years from the days when Muhammad made his journey from Mecca to Medina.)

Do you Know the Meaning of the Word Ephemeral?

Ephemeral: adj: lasting for a very short time – Oxford Little Dictionary

Soon as we begin to start to read and write as children, it is imposed on us that we should be on a lifelong quest to improve our vocabularies. And why not? The more words you know, the better you will be able to express yourself. The more you rely on words, the less you have to use gestures, facial expressions, and body language.

I used to look up words in the dictionary a lot when I was younger but then life gets in the way. You get busy and do not always care as much about adding words to your intellectual database.

Every once in a while, though, you come across a word that you want to look up the meaning of. Cell phones have made this so easy. You just type it in Google, and it gives you the meaning and pronunciation right away.

But as we all age, it also becomes easier to forget newly learned words. One proven way around that is to try and use any new word in a sentence right away and you are then unlikely to forget the word and hopefully it gets committed to your memory.

I came across one such word recently. Ephemeral. It is a nice-sounding word. A-fem-erel. Initially when I heard this word, I had a feeling that I knew its meaning but when I started trying to use it in my language, I realized that I actually didn't know its meaning and had never used it in my conversations or writings.

I looked it up and the description of the word in the dictionary was very straightforward – "*lasting for a very short time.*" It sounded like this word would be the antonym of "eternal." I liked the word and the meaning instantly and wanted it to be a part of my vocabulary, so I tried to use it in a sentence.

As I was racking my brain to make a sentence with the word Ephemeral in it, just like we were taught to do when we were in elementary school, life got in the way. My kids barged in and unapologetically broke my chain of thought and insisted that I drive them to the grocery store right away.

The next morning, as I was shuffling through my music playlists on Spotify to choose some nice and new music before I started my run, I came across this song which I had heard multiple times before but never paid attention to the lyrics.

This time I listened intently and realized that the song was about a number of things in life that are very precious but last for a very short period of time.

Suddenly, it clicked that the song was about "ephemeral" things in life, and I got excited that I had not forgotten the word and now it was a part of my vocabulary. I listened to the song and started enjoying all the ephemeral things mentioned in the song.

The song spoke about the raindrops that fall from the sky and land on leaves becoming dew drops. The same sun that gives them light to reflect and in doing so, they shine like beautiful diamonds, now dries them up with the heat as they disappear.

I looked around and as I was running by the canal, I could see the dew drops on the grass and the trees and enjoyed the song while it was playing. By the time my run came to an end, most of the dewdrops had evaporated. How ephemeral, I thought.

Ephemeral things in life

The song then spoke about the rays of sunlight that lighten up a courtyard in the midst of a brutal winter but then the evening sets in.

It spoke about those few moments of sleep when you are having a beautiful dream having a conversation with a deceased family member who is alive in the dream, but then you wake up realizing that they are gone. It spoke about a beautiful fragrance that is associated with a childhood memory, but you seldom encounter it anymore. It spoke about the feeling of your first crush when you are growing up which can hardly ever be duplicated again.

One of the topmost reasons for people to hate running is because they find it boring. This is exactly the reason why long-distance runners run. While you are at it, while the body has to toil mile after mile, the brain has nothing to do.

Unlike any other sport where you have to constantly be thinking about a certain maneuver or to win a point against an opponent, your mind while running doesn't have much to do.

At one point, a detachment happens between your mind and your body. This is the time when the mind drifts away, oblivious of the discomfort being signaled in from the body. The endorphins also kick in around the same time. This is when the mind starts thinking and goes on a very long tangent.

Soon not only your body is running but your mind also starts engaging in what seems like a long-distance thought process. This is when I started reflecting on all the ephemeral things in my own life.

Ahmet the Turkish Tailor

Just the day prior, I went to the dry cleaners to pick up my shirts. The owner is a Turkish guy, Ahmet. He is the kind of a guy who still takes cash and does not want to deal with bank cards or other forms of payment. If you are short on change, he tells you that you can pay the balance next time. He is neatly dressed and wears spectacles that visibly appear repaired from one end. He is about the same age as me, in his mid-forties. When he speaks, you feel like he is speaking from his heart. Simplicity is plastered over his face.

Once as I entered his store, he was finishing lunch and I asked him, "Who cooked this meal Ahmet? It smells nice!"

"My wife," he said. "But the best cook in the whole family is actually my mother-in-law. Here, try this, it's called a Dolma."

Having just finished my lunch, I politely declined but thought to myself, who does that anymore nowadays? Who offers you a dolma when you're picking up your laundry?

Anyways, this day, behind the counter there was a large poster of a young handsome teenager with a congratulatory salutation of "Graduate 2021" written just underneath his picture.

"This is my eldest son. He got accepted into college," he said with great pride. I congratulated him. While he was hand-writing a receipt for me, he thanked me but did not look up in my eyes. I got a bit puzzled but then he looked up and to my surprise, I saw tears in his eyes.

Thinking that he should be happy that his son graduated, I asked him what happened. "I'm sad. He wants to go away for college. I will miss him. He is still my little boy. Time went by so fast." How ephemeral his son's childhood must have seemed to him, I thought.

I had always thought of graduation as a happy event in life but now I wondered if it was actually a sad moment too. I attempted a consolatory remark along the lines of "you should be happy Ahmet that he is a responsible young man on his way to building a nice new life for himself and you should be such a proud father."

But now it was his turn to see my eyes well-up because my mind started to think about my own daughter who was just going to start her sophomore year in high school. She is beaming with the ambition to go to college and already dreaming about dorm life in big cities. I do not feel ready for her to leave me yet. But then perhaps, I never will be.

In the part of the world where I grew up, daughters live with their parents until they get married, and it is a very typical visual in movies as much as in real life where the father is crying at the time when the daughter gets married and goes to the house of her husband.

The trend is now shifting towards more girls getting educated and seeking local colleges resulting in daughters not leaving the house until a much older age. I thought that I would have to experience the moment of my daughter's separation just in another three years when she goes to college. I could try to convince her to get admission into a local college but how can I clip the wings of such an ambitious flight? But she was just born.

She was just learning to walk and talk. How could she grow up so fast? Why does she have to leave? How will I live without her? Why did her time living with me have to be so ephemeral? Not fair.

Some more ephemeral things in life

Mile after mile, I kept looking back at my life and thought about so many other ephemeral things of the past. My mind wandered to the time when we were kids in elementary school. A house filled with five brothers and our mom and dad.

We used to love going to school and used to wait every night until our dad came home, and we all sat at the dinner table.

At that time, as a child, I was naïve to think that this would always be the structure of my life, but it changed in its entirety with the passage of time without even realizing when and how it was changing.

If you think of your life in decades, you realize how your life becomes so different in each decade and makes you think how your remaining decades will be, which you have no control over.

We used to go to our maternal grandparents' house every Sunday for dinner. My aunts and uncles of varying ages would also get together. Our grandmother's cooking and our grandfather's hospitality were famous in the family.

At that time, we felt that these Sunday family dinners would be a permanent part of our lives. Even after my grandfather retired and perhaps his income dwindled, and my grandmother started aging, limiting her capacity to cook the large family dinners, the get-togethers continued on.

Then one day, when we came back from school, we saw our mom very anxious and tearful because my grandfather had had a heart attack. He remained hospitalized for a few days and eventually came back home.

On that Sunday, I still vaguely remember getting mentally ready to go for our big family dinner, but our mom told us that we will not be going. We didn't ask why, and she didn't explain either. That was the end of those Sunday dinners. How ephemeral, now that I think about it.

The unhelpful Eritrean Taxi Driver

I recently took the kids on a family trip to New York City. We had a lot of fun. On our way back, we took the cab home from the train station.

As I walked out of the station, with two large pieces of luggage dragging behind me, I saw a number of taxis parked right outside. It was extremely cold, and the wind chill was bitter. I made eye contact with the taxi driver who was standing first in line. He motioned to me that his taxi was available. Usually, at this point, the taxi drivers get down and help you with loading the luggage in the trunk. He did not show any signs of moving.

He lowered the window and asked me to put both pieces of luggage right next to him on the passenger seat. I asked him if he was sure because I did not want to ruin his seats. "Your luggage will be right next to me, and I will keep an eye on it." I rolled my eyes (when he was not looking) and put the heavy pieces on the front seat and asked the kids to get into the taxi.

I kept thinking about his discourteous behavior of not even getting out of the car to help me but then I argued with myself that it's not his job to haul luggage for me. I should be able to handle my own suitcases.

As we started driving towards our house, he started talking to us. He told us that he was from Eritrea and had lived in Rochester for about fifteen years which is about the same period of time I have also lived here. I told them that my kids who were accompanying me were both born in Rochester.

He told me that he was Muslim, and we both knew the Imam of our Islamic Center. He asked us where we were returning from. We told him that we had an amazing vacation in New York City. We enjoyed a musical and walked along the Brooklyn Bridge for the first time.

So far, the whole conversation was nothing but predictable small talk. Then he asked a question that changed the mood in the car. "And where is mommy?" He obviously did not know that we had divorced, and the kids' mother lived in another state. "She lives in Virginia," I said. He went silent for a few moments as if he did not know how to respond. He was clearly taken aback by our situation.

Finally he responded, "But kids this age cannot live without their mother?" This is when my daughter, who is growing into an intelligent young woman, stepped in, "No it's okay, this is the best arrangement for our family." This was a very polite way of saying, "We don't want your pity, we are managing well."

We continued small talk for the rest of the taxi ride. When our home arrived, I got down again thinking that he may help a little with unloading the luggage.

But this time again, he did not move out of his seat. I shrugged my shoulders and pulled out my heavy luggage from the passenger seat. Still feeling a bit awkward about our conversation in the car, I asked him how much money I owed him. As I was handing him over the cash, my eyes drifted towards him and now it was my turn to be taken aback. He had no legs!

He was driving the car using a metal device where he was able to press the gas and brake pedals with his hands. This solved the conundrum of why he wasn't getting down to help me with my luggage.

As a physician I feel comfortable asking people about their medical issues, so I asked, "How did you lose your legs?"

"Polio my friend. You don't see this disease anymore because of vaccines but a lot of kids lost their legs when I was a child," he replied.

"Oh yes, I know exactly what you're talking about. I have an aunt who has lost all function of her right arm because of polio," I replied.

As an attempt at commiseration, I continued. "It must be hard for you to make a living this way though."

This time, it was his moment to give me an "I don't need your pity" look and he replied, "No, thanks to God, I manage just fine."

This was only a short taxi ride home. A brief casual conversation. An ephemeral moment. But it reiterated an important lesson.

Everybody that we come across in life is going through their own struggles. They are on a journey to remain happy in the face of adversity. It is important to understand and respect that.

Lesson to be learnt from ephemeral things in life

The last thing I want to do is to leave you with the feeling that ephemeral is a negative word, an unwanted emotion. There has to be something good about this word too. It's quite similar in character to nostalgia, which is a tricky emotion. It makes you wonder whether it leaves you more sad or happy. Life is a constant struggle where happiness is achieved only if you can learn to live in the moment.

The present moment is all that was and all that will be. When we understand this fact, there will be nothing left to fear. But it is so difficult to live in the moment. The mind keeps wandering ahead or behind all the time. Some people constantly live in the past and cannot let go. Others are so focused on the future that their "today" is miserable.

One way of trying to live in the moment is to constantly look around and find the ephemeral things in life. If you look, you will find them. Lots of them. In fact, our whole existence is so ephemeral. The entire documented human history is only a few thousand years old. The size of our planet compared to the vastness of the universe is frighteningly miniscule.

In the midst of such an ephemeral existence, happiness is to live each ephemeral moment with such presence of mind and awareness, so as to make its beauty eternal. It is not easy to do, but it's worth trying, every once in a while.

Tell me About the Moment your Father Died

Friends get each other talking

I'm trying to remember how it came about. Some of my friends who have been friends for four decades, that is, since elementary school, but living in different parts of the world now, have come up with a routine. We talk by WhatsApp video chat every now and then.

One day, as we were talking freely, no judgments, only comfort and love, pulling each other's legs as soon as an opportunity arose.

All of a sudden one of us started talking about the moment that his father had died. Maybe it was the comfort level of talking to people who were closer to him in many ways more than his own family that he started sharing his innermost feelings with us.

I heard his story and thought for a moment how it must have been for him to go through his circumstances at the moment of his father's death. I wanted to say something in return to make him feel better. I wanted to comfort him, console him, and tell him that I was there for him. But I could not come up with a good way of expressing my support.

Anything I would say would sound so superficial and artificial.

How could I convey my feelings to him in a way that he understood my desire to comfort him? My mind went blank. But then it came to me. I would share with him the story of the moment my father died. That would be the best way to express my true emotion towards him.

It's hard to talk about your parent's death

Some people who are reading this will be fortunate in that their parents may still be alive. May God give them longevity brimming with good health. You are the people who live with the fear of seeing a day when your parents will die. I tell you; it's not a good day.

But it will pass, like all other things in life. But those of us who have lost a Dad or a Mom or a Baba or Amma or Abu or Ami; you will not disagree with me if I say that it was probably one of the worst days of your life. We often push our worst feelings and memories towards the rear of our minds. Shove them somewhere, where you hope to not see them again but know that they will keep coming back because there is no way of getting rid of them.

But one way of making these feelings more tolerable is to keep invoking them again and again. Do you know that if you are allergic to something, the doctors repeatedly expose you to the same stimulus to "sensitize" your body so that you can be exposed to it and not get the allergic reaction anymore?

Similarly, if you recall your ugly memories often, they don't remain that ugly anymore. And on top of that, if you start expressing those feelings, it ends up being cathartic. I learned the meaning of the word "cathartic" after a very long time.

It's a release. It's closure. It is therapy. If you keep your feelings and emotions inside, they pent up and start creating pressure in your head just like a pot of water when it is being boiled.

As soon as you express those feelings, and put them into words, either by saying or writing, you release that pressure inside your head. It is liberating.

In the same way, I would ask you to recall the moment that your parent died. Do not put that memory on the back burner. Express it and notice that memory turning from a bitter memory into a sweet memory. It will become sweet because you shared it with your loved ones and now you are not the only one to bear the burden of that memory. You have shared the weight with others, and it has become easier to carry the memory.

The subtlety of the signs of the onset of dementia

When I think about my father, the very first word that comes to my mind is: "nice guy." It's funny to think of your father as that but that's really who he was. Easy going, lenient, understanding, always trying to make a lame joke. Proud of the fact that he worked hard and was a simple, uncomplicated, and self-made man.

His cognitive decline came at a time when he was at the pinnacle of his intellectual accomplishments. He was the Dean of the Post Graduate Medical Institute at that time. That can be considered as the highest level of academic medicine to achieve in this profession.

The onset of dementia is usually not abrupt and can be slow. It seeps into your personality gradually so as not to be able to remember a specific moment of onset.

But when you look back, you realize that some events were the beginnings of the shortcomings of mental capacities.

He always raised us very tight with money. My brothers and I often joke that he gives us enough money to fulfill our needs, but we never had enough to party or be extravagant or wasteful.

We figured that something was wrong when he started giving us the amount of money we asked him for. We did not know at that time that he had started losing the capability of doing the math when dealing with money, but we could not understand at that time. We were just happy that he was giving us the money.

He started making mistakes while tipping. Giving a much higher or a lower amount compared to the 20% that he meticulously taught us to calculate in our heads while we were growing up.

My mother recalls that while he was traveling with her during Hajj, he was a different man. She still cannot put a finger on how he was different but being someone who lived with that man for the last three decades and knowing him inside and out, she could feel the difference. Something had happened.

His routine had changed. His thought process was different. But she did not yet know what misery this change was a sign for, that he and the whole family would have to endure for the next decade or so.

It is not uncommon to see elderly people in their eighties or nineties be moderately demented. In fact, it is considered normal by many to "lose it" with age. But developing signs of dementia in one's sixties and then progressing on to end-stage within a few years is uncommon and particularly devastating.

My father's cognitive decline proceeded with a snail's pace but what appeared to us as lightning speed. Every year was worse than the prior.

We did not even know what was going on for the first few years. We knew something was different, but we could not tell that this was something pathological. The signs started becoming clearer, unfortunately. We all used to wait for him to come home to have dinner.

I don't remember a single day of my childhood where we may have proceeded with having dinner without waiting for his arrival back from work. One day he came home much later than the usual time. This was not the time of cell phones. You would not go crazy with frantic phone calls and texts if somebody was a few minutes late. You would wait. When he finally arrived home, he had a confused and slightly embarrassed look on his face.

When my mother asked him the reason for being late, he told her that for some reason he could not find his way back home and he was roaming around in the neighborhood for a while. Again, we did not think much of it at that time.

A few years later, I had moved to the United States and my parents visited us when we were expecting the birth of my daughter, their first grandchild and the only girl in two generations.

We are all brothers, and we do not have a sister, so the birth of a girl had an extra significance and excitement.

My father used to take care of all travel-related tasks such as keeping the tickets and passports safe in his coat pocket, checking in at the airline counter and carrying the boarding passes, and figuring out which carousel the baggage will arrive at.

Now he had lost his sharpness, and my mother had to gradually start taking over these tasks. My mother knew something was not right, but she could not put a finger on it.

Son breaking the diagnosis of dementia to dad, both physicians

I had started my medical training and had started seeing patients with dementia. I was having a conversation with my dad one day about our mutual profession of medicine.

Here he was, a seasoned pediatrician and I was a budding internist, a dad and son having an exchange about our beloved profession.

I would often ask him questions to which he would give me guidance and practical answers. All of a sudden it popped into my mind to ask him whether the change in his behavior that my mother was noticing could be the beginnings of a diagnosis of dementia? He did not have a response to that.

I could sense the genuine expression of not knowing the answer on his face. I am still not sure if it was because he did not know the clinical presentation of dementia (because he, although was an experienced clinician but was a pediatrician and this is a disease of the elderly) or whether it was because he did not have insight into his illness just as most patients with dementia don't.

I took him to a local neuropsychiatrist and also discussed his case with the Professor who I was working with those days. I still remember that after listening to me go on about his symptoms for a while, his only answer in the end to me was, "I'm sorry to hear that about your father Farhan." I was expecting him to offer some advice, some tests, and treatments but he did not offer any. The finality of his statement struck me.

Not only had he confirmed the diagnosis but had also indicated to me that there weren't any effective treatments available. My eyes welled up but could not prepare me enough for the treacherous journey that lay ahead.

I can still remember the day when my mother and I were sitting in the waiting room in the doctor's office. He had taken my father into the room by himself to ask him questions which he was supposed to answer without our help.

Earlier we had witnessed the man who had the largest clinical practice in town, mentally reduced to being unable to copy a simple picture of a house that preschoolers usually draw easily.

We grew up with his stories of how he was proud that he always scored a hundred in his math exam and was now unable to subtract sevens serially out of a hundred. I started lecturing my mother how she now had to take over the finances and all other such dealings of the family.

His love for his time in America:

He had trained in the United States and was amongst the few people who relocated back to their country. He had the most fulfilling career in Pakistan with tremendous achievements both academically and financially. He could probably never have achieved this kind of success if he had stayed back in the United States. But his heart always spoke about America with love and fondness.

He was asked by his brother and father-in-law to stay in Pakistan which he did, but in his wishful moments, he would always reminisce about his time in America.

When I told him that I had decided to pursue medical education in the United States, he seemed genuinely happy for me. When I was applying for residency positions and was wondering which hospitals to apply to, he used to say, "every hospital in America is the best hospital in the world."

When he was in the United States, he had the opportunity to become a citizen but at that time, acquiring US citizenship was not such a big deal.

For him, it was a matter of just filling out a form and putting it into the mail, but he decided not to, primarily because it would have been one more form to fill.

Later the world events changed in a way that even obtaining a visa to visit the country became quite difficult, let alone obtaining citizenship.

When I got my Green Card (permanent residence), I was on my way to work and called up my father. He had lost his capacity to understand the meaning of naturalization but somewhere buried in his mind was to congratulate me. "I'm proud of you" was what he said.

Perhaps he figured that whatever I had achieved in the medical profession, he had already achieved it but since I also obtained the citizenship of his beloved country, I had done something that he did not do and hence was proud of me.

Another time he was visiting me; he had started to become more childlike. In the morning I would fill a bowl of cheerios with fresh cold milk that he would love to have. He loved fresh milk to drink taken directly from the fridge and without adding anything into it.

In fact, that is what he would bring us to drink the first thing in the morning when he used to wake us up for school. He would enjoy his cheerios like a school child.

In the evening, I would put a chair in our driveway, and he would just sit there and stare at the front yard and the passing cars and say nothing.

When you said something to him, instead of being able to come up with meaningful responses, he would just smile and if he saw you laughing, he would laugh with you. He was happily demented. His recollection of America was that of the busy life of New York City where he had spent most of his time in his youth.

Now he was visiting my place, which was a ranch house in suburban America and was nothing like New York City. He was pleasantly confused about that and would often say, "Is this the same America? Is there another America as well?"

When the dementia is not so subtle anymore

I did not live with him for the last several years of his life. He was in Pakistan, and I was in the United States. My mother and younger brothers lived with him through his entire journey from the diagnosis of dementia until his death. They have a thousand more stories to tell than I do.

But I do remember every few months, hearing a new story of something embarrassing happening in front of other people that my mother would tell me about. He could not recognize her anymore. He behaved as if she was some "lady" living in the house.

He also stopped recognizing my brothers. He would behave very formally with them like you do when a distant acquaintance is visiting you after a long time.

He could not work anymore. Patients would still come to him because of his fame as a pediatrician but he did not have the capability of practicing medicine anymore. If these capacities were lost relatively quickly, it would have been easier for him to stop working but the cognitive decline was so slow and subtle that it became difficult to decide when to ask him to stop working.

His colleagues would 'cover up' for his decline by having other doctors make clinical decisions in case he was not making the right decisions, but his practice managers still would not let him stop working because his name was selling. I had a deep conflict with that practice, but I was thousands of miles away and could not put an end to that practice because

I was told that I lived in a different world and that they had their own way of handling things.

Eventually, he was not even able to put up a show of being a physician in front of the patients and his practice was taken over by his junior colleagues.

Phone call from mom, "It's time to come home"

One day I received a call from my mom. I was moonlighting in a smaller hospital close to West Virginia. I had just begun my fellowship in Oncology at Georgetown University. It was not unusual for my mom to call me and tell me how my father was doing and to obtain medical advice. This time her tone was different.

She had seen or experienced something that had invoked the sense in her that he did not have too much time left to live. She said, "Come home. Your father is not doing well. I have also asked Salman (my older brother who was also overseas) to just come."

When you live so far away from home, every phone call about an ailing family member becomes a source of anxiety. It becomes hard to decide when to pack up your bags, leave your life as is ongoing, and head back home.

If there is one tragic event, the decision of whether to go or not becomes easy but if somebody is suffering from a chronic illness, with periodic exacerbations, it is hard to decide when to go. This time it was not hard to figure out though because of the clarity in my mother's voice.

I walked in the very next day into my boss's office and told him the situation. Fortunately, I work in a profession where we are helping people in similar situations on a daily basis. I started explaining my father's situation to him but the great man that he was, stopped me mid-sentence and said, "Your dad is dying? Go. Go home."

I again started to ask him about who would cover for me and some other logistics of my vacation, but he did not let me finish what I wanted to say and asked me to just go and tend to my family. He would take care of how to handle the workload of my absence. Needless to say that I will remain forever grateful to that man.

The dying days

When I reached Peshawar, instead of going home from the airport, I headed directly to the hospital. My dad was surrounded by family and friends. I started looking at his medical chart and examined him and realized that there was nothing acute going on. It was rather a situation where nobody at home was equipped to deal with his worsening chronic medical issues. I conferred with my brothers, and we brought him home.

Hospice care is non-existent in Pakistan, so we had to handle everything on our own. We hired a nurse who had absolutely no medical training but was supposed to be with my father at all times and help him with all activities of daily living ranging from feeding him to helping him use the bathroom.

He had a lot of secretions in his throat on which he would start choking. We brought a suction machine for which we would take turns to suck the secretions out of his throat. This would irritate his throat to the point that blood would start coming out. This is also when I realized how difficult it is to be a doctor or a nurse for your own family member.

Too much love or hate can impair your medical judgment. There were times that while suctioning him, if he started screaming in pain or started choking, I would have to stop because I would start crying myself. This is also where I realized the importance of professionals taking care of people who are towards the end of their life.

I was in close touch with the Palliative care professors at Georgetown via email. I would ask questions about how to handle any of the situations at the bedside in my father's final days.

Finding well-trained palliative care doctors and hospice nurses is impossible in Peshawar. We knew everybody in the medical community since we belonged to it but the medical expertise of how to take care of a person at the end of his life was simply not available. We had to do everything on our own. By this time, I had good training in these issues, but it was hard for me to apply my medical knowledge to my own father's care.

You cannot be your own dad's doctor

When his secretions became too much, choking him every few hours, I asked the nurse to cut down on the liquid feeds that we were giving him through the tube that went directly into his stomach. When my mother found it, she was livid. "Keep your training to yourself, I will not let you starve your father to death!"

When my father was in intense pain, which became apparent by how hard he was clenching his teeth and tightening his fists, I tried to acquire strong pain medications for him which could be given to him intravenously since he was not able to swallow pills.

I called one of his students who himself was a Professor of Pediatrics, having no experience in adult end-of-life care, and asked him where I could find intravenous morphine. The response was, "he is also like a father to me, how can you even think about euthanizing him?" I realized that my expert medical training would not come to much use because of the complex cultural issues at hand.

The family wedding predicament

In the days when my father was totally incapacitated, we as a family had to make another big decision. My younger brother was supposed to get married.

The invitation cards had been sent out a few weeks prior. The venue was booked. All the food catering orders were finalized. It was supposed to be a big wedding with a large number of guests like many Pakistani weddings are.

As the date approached near, we became increasingly uneasy about whether we should go ahead with the wedding as planned or not.

Weddings are supposed to be happy events with joy and dancing and laughter and here we were, sad and our hearts crying every day looking at the state our father was in. How could we be hosting people with smiles on our faces when our father was suffering from pain and agony? There was talk about postponing the wedding. There were concerns brought up that it wouldn't look appropriate that our father is dying, and we are out there having a good time.

This is where my experience of working with my own patients' families helped. We are often asked by families about personal issues like when to travel or when to hold certain family events if a patient is dying.

I suggested that we go ahead with the wedding because if we didn't, it would feel as if we were waiting for our father to die so that we could move on with our lives. Also, we did not know how long he had left. In Pakistani culture, the girl's family would not want to wait that long.

Finally, we decided to move forward with the wedding. I can still remember telling my dad's nurse on the evening of the wedding, on my way to the wedding hall, to call only me or another brother in case my dad died while we were at the event.

We had a plan to keep it to ourselves and not let anyone know because we did not want a wedding ceremony to convert into a funeral. We would keep it hush until the next morning or so and then move on with the burial. God was kind to us and the wedding went on smoothly, without any hiccups.

When he was dying, and I had to leave

Being an immigrant to another country is not easy. One of the problems is that you are living so far away that it is not always possible to be at important family events such as the death of your own father. I had taken a few weeks off to be at my father's bedside.

My colleagues were very understanding of my situation especially when this is exactly the work we all do for a living, helping people and their families towards the end of their lives. I had not been asked to come back to work at any particular time.

But after spending about four weeks, I felt the burden of duty and decided to go back to work. I would not take advantage of their niceness by staying away from work for an extended period of time.

I could have easily taken another couple of weeks off, but we did not know how much longer my father had to live. It could be two weeks or two months. That is when I decided to fly back to the United States and go back to work.

As I saw my father for the last time and I turned around to leave, I had full realization that this was the last time I was seeing him alive.

The man that he was, was gone several years ago, his cognition and his personality robbed by dementia, but the physical body was also on its way out of this world.

My mother was standing there and I burst into tears with the intensity of a child. I'm used to giving advice, even to my parents in any situation and while I was sobbing, I remember telling my mom to bury my dad in our ancestral graveyard in Charsadda which my dad always spoke about because that's where his dad was buried.

I flew back to Washington DC and resumed my job. My wife and kids were still in Pakistan. I was alone.

About a week later, one evening, I got a call from my brother who was a medical student at that time telling me that my father's blood pressure was quite low. They were smelling a very foul odor from his secretions, and it looked like a bad pneumonia was setting in, making him go into sepsis which is how an infection takes your life.

It was an indication that he did not have much time left. We agreed that we would just keep him comfortable and not take him to the hospital. I went to sleep.

The moment of his death

I woke up with a phone call from Pakistan. It has been fully erased from my memory of who called me, probably because of the shocking nature of the moment, but I was told that my father had died.

I was expecting a phone call like this for several months now which I thought would have prepared me for the moment when I will hear of his passing. Apparently, I wasn't.

This was the moment that is the most dreaded moment of anybody's entire life. The moment you hear or you see your father dying. I ended the conversation abruptly and hung up.

The moment I hung up, sitting up in my bed, a deep wail came from inside of my stomach and I burst out into a loud cry. I wept with such intensity that I did not think I was capable of. My clothes and the bed sheets were wet with my tears. There was nobody there to console me.

But I did not want anyone there anyway. I sat still for a few minutes. Then I got up, got ready, and went to work. I did not tell anyone at work that my father had died that morning. I did not want people to come and offer me their condolences because that would make me emotional. They would ask me to go home and take the day off. "Who works on the day their father dies," they would say. But what would I do if I went home?

There was nobody at home. I may not have been able to handle the loneliness. I was better off surrounded by people who did not know what was going on. Work was the best distraction under those circumstances.

I keep saying that being an immigrant is not easy. If you hear about a loved one's death, even if you catch the very next plane to be able to attend the funeral, it might take a good two to three days, between the long travel and the time zone difference, for you to reach there.

In the Islamic tradition, embalming the body and keeping it in the morgue for prolonged periods of time are discouraged. The burial should take place promptly, the sooner the better. I had just returned after spending a month with my father and even if I decided to go back to attend the funeral, I simply could not make it.

This way, like millions of other immigrants, I could not go through the experience of burying my father.

The profound act of burial

There is a certain feeling of closure that is associated with spending time with the dead body of your loved one. When you see them lifeless, not breathing, body as still as an inanimate object; the reality of this existence strikes you. You mourn until you tire out.

If you think of it, you are a biological product of that person and when you perform the final rites such as washing the body and covering it in drapes, preparing for the burial, it is as if you are laying to rest a part of your own body, your own existence.

As you lower the body into the ground and cover it with earth, your mind goes into a state of void and emptiness where there is no room for any worldly thoughts.

When you finally walk away from the grave, issues of life start seeping back into your mind. For a while, you push those thoughts away but slowly, they keep coming back to the forefront, eventually helping you overcome the great loss. If you are unable to participate in the burial of your loved one, you are deprived of going through all these emotions.

The other most common way in which humans bid farewell to the bodies of their loved ones is cremation. I have never participated in a cremation ceremony so I cannot attest to the emotions that one goes through while this is happening.

But I have heard about the sentimental value that is attached to the ashes and how these are handled by different people and cultures.

Humans have developed different ways of doing things and it is not uncommon for people to frown upon and criticize other groups' practices and rituals. For example, I have often heard people speak with disgust about some cultures that place the corpses on tall towers to be eaten by vultures.

At one point I also thought of this as a barbaric practice but then somewhere I read that the philosophy behind this practice is that those cultures want to be beneficial to Mother Earth even in their death. The vultures that eat the corpses are also God's creation and those humans, even in their death, are providing sustenance to the birds. If you think of it this way, you can appreciate rather than abhor this practice.

After death, our parents live through us

It has been about a decade since my father died. But I feel that he has been gone for two decades because his cognition started waning long before his physical body left us. Life moves on. Bearing the loss of his death becomes easy by remembering his own words.

Anytime a tragic event would happen in our lives, he would just say, "this is a part of life." I don't feel sad when I think about him. I always feel happy. I never wished that he had lived longer. I feel that this was his destiny. How can I challenge destiny? Who am I to challenge God?

I still see him in my dreams every few months. I have dreamt that we are sitting together, and his cognition is back. I'm telling him about how he lost all his mental capabilities and how difficult it was to handle everything. He listens and sympathizes and for a moment, in the dream, while sitting with him, I feel that his protracted illness and dementia was nothing but a bad dream, but then I wake up realizing that every single bit of it was a raw truth. I feel that he lives through me. Through my brothers.

Often when a brother speaks or makes a certain gesture, it is just like my dad's. Some of my own habits, simple things like how I touch the side of my teeth with my tongue, how I cross my legs while relaxing, how I like to wear my cozy robe and socks at home, my thin shoulders and awkwardly protruding belly; are all reminders that he is still living through me.

With the advent of cellphone cameras, we now take a generous number of pictures even of the littlest things in life. There was a time when you had a film in the camera that would take only thirty-two pictures, and you had to think so many times before taking a picture.

Now you see, pictures of deceased people are circulated on social media as common practice. Some religions and cultures frown upon it but it still does not stop people from taking these pictures and sharing them. Social media has seeped into our existence like water through a crack.

Since I could not be at my father's funeral, my mom asked me if I wanted her to send a picture of his face after passing away since that is probably what others had started doing. Maybe some people even participate in funerals and burials by FaceTime. I shuddered at this thought. I immediately refused. I don't know what made me decline this offer instantly without even putting any thought into it.

This was my chance to participate in the last rites of my dad and could provide me some closure. But now that I think of it, I simply did not have the guts to see him like that.

When I visited Pakistan, I went to his grave. It was a nice way to pay respect but just looking at a tombstone with his name and scripture inscribed on it, did not do too much to stir emotions. It is also possible that I remained relatively unemotional at that time because I was used to grieving alone, by myself.

Perhaps I was surrounded by people who accompanied me to the cemetery, and I was victim to the ultimate curse of human thinking called, "what will people say." I was not letting my emotions be expressed freely and was inadvertently suppressing them.

I would still say that visiting a loved one's grave has its special significance but the true way of remembering someone is by talking about them.

Often when I'm talking to my children, I interject my father's words into conversations. Of course, it is not pleasant to talk about the dying moments of your parents, but it is important to recall these details every once in a while, and to put them into words.

This is what brings you closer to the people with whom you are sharing the memory of these moments.

I encourage you to remember the moments you experienced when your father died and share them with someone. If your father is alive, may he live a long, happy and healthy life. Amen.

The Slow and Painful Death of Handwriting

It was a particularly busy day at work. I moved between patients quickly, making sure that I did not appear rushed and trying to give each patient the time and attention they deserved. The email inbox was overflowing, and the phone calls were relentlessly interrupting.

The secretary reluctantly walked into my office, perhaps worrying that I might snap at her if she piled another task on my desk. She waited until I got off the phone. "Here are some disability forms. I have already filled them out. You just need to sign and date at the bottom," she said.

That was easy enough for me, so a brief sense of relief came over me, reflected by my facial expressions.

The next moment, something happened that made me feel like my life had changed in a way I had never expected. My hands went to the front pocket of my shirt and then to the inside pocket of my jacket, and I could not find a pen. I quickly turned to the corner of my desk where all the stationery was supposed to be, and I realized that there was no pen there either.

A strange sense of sadness and embarrassment overcame me because I was neck-deep in the middle of a busy workday and did not have a pen. A similar feeling that a warrior would have thousands of years ago stranded in the middle of a battleground and not being able to find his sword.

I asked the secretary if she had a pen, and she rushed to her desk and brought me a ballpoint pen with which I signed the document and moved on to dictate my next patient note. For many, this may not be a big deal at all, but for me, this moment represented the end of an era in human history.

My memory goes back to kindergarten when my parents brought me a four-lined notebook, which helped me learn how to write. In Elementary (Junior) school, we were only allowed to write with a pencil. I don't know the exact reason behind not allowing elementary school children to use a pen. Maybe it was because they did not want little children to make a mess with the ink pens.

Perhaps somebody decided that using a pencil might be better for developing a child's handwriting skills. Whatever the reason, it was one of my biggest excitements as a child to graduate to Middle (Senior) school, where we were allowed to use ink pens for the first time.

There was another rule here, though. Only fountain pens were allowed, and ballpoint pens could not be used. Again, I do not understand the reason behind this rule, but we always thought this would be better for handwriting development.

Some kids started using ballpoint pens instead of fountain pens towards the later years of high school, and the teachers did not restrict them from doing so, but some of us continued to use the fountain pens since we had gotten so used to it.

Also, it had been built up in our psyche that any official handwriting should be done with the fountain pen. Just like you would always wear a tie and a jacket instead of jeans and a T-shirt to a job interview, you would also write an official letter with a fountain pen in blue or black ink instead of writing with a ballpoint pen in any other color.

My generation, which is people born in the latter part of the twentieth century, has witnessed the transformation of the world within our lifetime, perhaps as no other generation has seen in the past.

It feels that the progress made in the digitalization of the world over the last few decades would otherwise have been expected to take place over centuries.

We went from having one rotary-dial phone in the whole house to a smartphone carried by every member of the family. We went from finding our way using cumbersome road maps and stopping at each gas station to ask for directions to following satellite-controlled navigation systems that gave us accurate directions and even the estimated time of arrival at a particular destination.

When we were kids, our uncle lived overseas, and I can remember it being a big family event for him to call us. He would place a three-minute call through an operator, which probably cost him a fortune, and only my grandparents were allowed to talk to him due to the limited time that they had. We would all still gather around the phone and enjoy the call by listening to our side of the conversation.

Now, every morning, on my way to work, I press one button on my phone, and I am not only able to talk but also to have a video chat with my mom and my brothers at the same time while we all live in different parts of the world in different time zones.

Today, a child learns to use the keyboard before learning to hold a pencil. That was not the case just a decade earlier. When we were kids, nobody knew or was expected to know how to use a keyboard.

You only needed to learn how to type if you wanted to become a stenographer or an office secretary.

When we were kids, we used to love going to our father's office during summer break and hanging out in his office while he was doing his work. We loved to explore his drawers and use his office stationery to write with. We loved sitting at his official desk and chair and having access to refreshments in the fridge.

There was an extra typewriter in his office that was not being used much, and I had asked his secretary to give me a few typing lessons, where he showed me which fingers to use for certain alphabets on the keyboard.

It was much harder to type on a typewriter than on a computer keyboard since those keys were weighted and much harder to press, especially the alphabets that had to be typed with the ring and little fingers. This is a similar difference when you play the weighted keys of a piano versus a digital keyboard.

My brothers were spending all their time playing endless hours of video games on Atari and Nintendo while I was learning to type on a Typewriter. They made fun of me and thought I was a nerd and wasting my time, and I felt the same way about them.

It turned out that handwriting would be replaced mainly by typing no matter what kind of work you do.

It is nice to think of people as parts of certain arbitrarily defined generations when it comes to discussing topics like this. The baby boomers are people who were born in the 1940s to 1960s. Then came the generations X, Y, and Z. Generation X, to which I belong, comprises the people born between the 1960s and 1980.

Next in line is Generation Y, also known as the "Millennials," who are people born between 1980 and 1995. The latest is Generation Z, which is the kids born after the year 1995. I have noticed that most Millennials may never even have used a fountain pen, and they do not understand its different parts and how to hold or write with it.

Humans have probably been writing ever since Homo sapiens cognition developed. Maybe when writing on the walls of the caves, man used sharp objects or natural materials to etch or engrave on stone. Then came the use of papyrus and other natural materials, such as bamboo or animal hides, to write on.

The first use of paper has been described in China as early as a few hundred years BC. For centuries, the pens used to write would not carry any ink but had to be dipped in little inkpots. This was messy with ink stains on hands and paper and cumbersome with having to dip the nib in the inkpot repeatedly, breaking the natural flow of handwriting.

The first mention of a fountain pen documented in history is from 974 AD, when an Egyptian King desired a pen to be made that would carry the ink in it rather than having to dip it into the inkpot repeatedly.

Later in history, the fountain pen was mentioned during Europe's 15th and 16th century Renaissance period. The handwriting of Leonardo Da Vinci has been analyzed, and experts have concluded that some may have been written with fountain pens.

By the mid-19th century, different pen designers had started obtaining patents for their fountain pens, and some of the noteworthy names were those of John Scheffer and John Jacob Parker.

These pens now contained a reservoir in which one could draw a reasonable amount of ink and keep writing for several pages without having to refill. The ink would pass from the reservoir to the nib using the principles of gravity and capillary action. It wasn't until the early twentieth century that the "Ball Pen" (ballpoint pen) was invented.

These pens were further improvised so that instead of a nib, there was a tiny ball made of metal such as brass, steel, or tungsten. The ink was also improvised to be more viscous, less likely to smudge on the paper, and would dry quickly.

This ink could be carried in the reservoir and used for a significantly longer time to the point that the modern ballpoint pen can write for thousands of pages without needing to refill the ink.

With the mass production of these ball pens came affordability, and these pens could be made at such a low cost that one could easily use a pen and throw it away once the ink was finished.

When I was in Middle school in the 1980s, we would buy very affordable fountain pens at our school bookstore. These came with reservoirs, which we would fill with ink sold in small bottles. We would have to refill the ink once every few hours or days, depending on how much we wrote.

Later, pre-filled ink cartridges became available, but these were not the most cost-effective since they were more expensive and had to be thrown away after each use. One ink bottle could perform the job of hundreds of pre-filled cartridges. Some kids still liked to use the pre-filled cartridges.

Still, once they ran out, instead of throwing them away, they would use a medical syringe to inject ink back into the cartridges to re-use them, which, of course, was not a very practical solution, and one was better off just buying ink bottles.

Our school mandated that we use blue ink. Later in high school, they allowed black ink, but many kids continued to use blue ink. Red ink was supposed to be used only by the teachers to mark our work, make corrections, and award grades. Our exams then did not have "multiple-choice questions".

Instead, we had to write essays and paragraphs as answers to all questions. The year-end exams were typically over three hours for each subject of study. We were given blank papers as answer sheets, usually with about 12 or 16 sheets of paper.

Although the teachers told us that the quality of our answers mattered rather than the quantity, it was an unspoken rule that the more you wrote, the better grade you would get. That would make one ask for additional sheets of paper if you had already used up the provided answer sheets. This would even be a competitive scenario when, hardly 30 minutes into a 3-hour exam, the first student who would raise a hand for an extra sheet of paper would look around the classroom with a conquering expression on their face.

Some of the best students would ask for several additional sheets that were even higher than the original answer sheet provided.

Finally, small pieces of thread were distributed to tie all the sheets together. This had to be done as neatly as possible. Teachers were more likely to give extra reward to the more voluminous answer sheets.

Another trick I used was to write the essays in black ink instead of blue ink and to write the headings in blue ink. This would make my answer sheet stand out among others, which was another way to convey to the teachers that my work was different and that I was looking for a better grade not only with the use of content but also additional credit for the presentation. It turned out that this strategy applies to everything in life.

No matter what job you do, there is one thing to be knowledgeable and competent at what you do, but what makes you stand out among your peers is how you present and deliver your work.

Handwriting and the use of Fountain Pens also became part of our identity and childhood memories. You would always recognize the handwriting of a classmate just like you would recognize their voice, laugh, or any other personal attribute.

If you were to find a piece of paper or notebook with no name written on it, you would easily guess who it belonged to by recognizing the handwriting, or you just had to ask around. One would also know who had good handwriting and who wrote illegibly.

Some kids had such lovely and neat handwriting that their notebooks would circulate in the whole class if any passages needed to be copied. One of the best comments was given by a teacher to my older brother when she said in front of the whole class that his handwriting reminded her of "pearls beautifully arranged on a necklace."

The neat kids kept their ink bottles clean and secure and kept a small piece of tissue paper nicely tucked inside the box to wipe away any smudges and spills quickly.

On the other hand, it was not unusual to see blue stains on the white shirts of the clumsy kids who could not handle the pens and the ink bottles very well.

You were never supposed to lend your favorite fountain pen to somebody else if they asked for it because, with months and sometimes years of writing, the nib would adapt to the slight pressure and slant of your handwriting. If somebody else wrote with it, they could ruin the subtle fineness of the nib.

The graduation day from high school used to be a big event. There were so many different ways to celebrate it. Some of those ways were, unfortunately, not very civil.

Some kids would fill their fountain pens with ink and flick them toward other kids, splashing ink on their clothes and leaving stains.

This practice was, of course, highly discouraged by the teachers, but still, things would go out of hand on the last day of school. One of my best friends and I were once caught splashing ink on each other, which, as you can imagine, was not difficult to get caught when your crisp white school shirt had multiple ink stains on it.

We were taken to the principal and were given the worst imaginable punishment. Our shirts were taken away, and we were made to stand shirtless in front of the whole school in a prominent location. This was an age when one was constantly trying to seek the opposite gender's attention and attraction.

When you had to stand shirtless with an unappealing skinny physique in front of the whole school, the incident ended up being high on the list of the most embarrassing moments of our lives. We laugh about it now but would not wish something like that to happen even to our worst enemies.

During medical school, our exams were conducted similarly to those in high school; we had to write essays in answer sheets. The same handwriting habits we had learned in school were used at this time without giving it too much thought.

Many students had started using ballpoint pens instead of fountain pens due to their ease of use, low cost, and maintenance.

After medical school, I started taking international exams to be licensed to train in the United States. This was the first time I took exams on a computer by clicking on the answers to multiple-choice questions without having to write anything on paper.

Later, when I started working as a physician, handwriting was still the way of documentation until the advent of electronic health records.

If you find any medical literature from a few decades or centuries ago, you will find that these patient notes were written in a very personable manner.

The doctors would describe the patients and their ailments using a literary style and human attributes of sympathy, empathy, intrigue, and even humor.

Later, with the increase of litigation and lack of time, the medical progress notes became more objective and "mechanical," which lacked documentation of the treating physician's personal feelings and focused more on creating a document that could be used as a legal record and not to put anything in there that could be used against the writer should the matter be taken up in the court of law.

The earliest electronic health record came in the 1960s but was not widely available or adaptable.

The United States government started using an early form of electronic health record at the Veteran's Affairs health facilities. In the 1990s, the internet gained widespread acceptance, and electronic health records became more mainstream.

However, it was later, in 2009, when laws were passed to transition the whole country's health care system to electronic records.

Using this legislation, doctors and hospitals were given higher payments if they transitioned to electronic health records.

However, this left them with no choice but to transition because if they preferred to use their old method of handwriting the medical records, they were indirectly penalized by lower reimbursements.

For doctors who had been in practice for decades, it was a huge undertaking, and they were faced with a choice of either retiring early or unwillingly and begrudgingly transitioning to the electronic method of keeping the health record.

Undoubtedly, electronic health records have significantly improved the ease of documentation and writing orders and the availability of such records at the palm of doctors' and patients' hands.

When on call, I can review a patient's chart from my smartphone and even place orders without getting out of bed. The patients receive their test results instantly and have direct access to their health records instantly from anywhere in the world.

But it is not as straightforward as it seems. There are significant downsides to electronic health records as well. It still ends up being a lively debate whether the medical care a patient receives has improved because of transitioning to the electronic health record.

Doctors are now spending most of their time documenting in the electronic record. This has taken away from a doctor's time with the patient. The history-taking and physical examination skills of physicians are becoming poorer. The sacred patient-doctor relationship is becoming weaker.

I wouldn't be surprised if, in the next couple of decades, doctors are just sitting at pharmacies or their homes and evaluating patients just by being given data from the computers and providing advice in the same way, never having laid a hand on a patient.

A doctor may only have to see a patient physically if a hands-on procedure has to be performed, such as surgery, endoscopy, etc. Ultimately, the patients will get the care they need, but we will not know health care as it has been known for centuries.

The image of a doctor will be replaced from one of a caring and thoughtful individual sitting at the bedside, holding the hand of an ailing patient, to a robotic human sitting endlessly in front of a computer screen.

Even today, in the United States of America, doctors spend probably 90 percent of their time sitting in front of the computer screen rather than at the patient's bedside.

If anybody wants to challenge that statistic, you are welcome to come and spend a day at work with me.

During my late 20s and 30s, I was newly married and had young kids. I was also going through my residency training, which involved long hours. I did not care much about what pen I would write with.

Many pharmaceutical companies typically provided ball pens, always available everywhere in the hospital. Then, during my 40s, I started to cherish things I used to like when I was younger. I rediscovered the music albums I loved during my teenage years. I watched some of my favorite movies again and read the books I liked in my younger years. This is when I realized I still liked to write with a fountain pen and wanted to try it again.

I went to Staples, which is the largest stationery store in America. To my surprise, while they had hundreds of different types of ballpoint pens, gel-ink pens and markers available, they had only one or two types of fountain pens, which came only with pre-filled ink cartridges.

I started asking around and researching the internet, where I could find a larger variety of Fountain Pens. I could only find one or two stores in major cities, such as New York or Washington DC, that sold fountain pens.

Somebody told me about a shop at a local mall where they had seen a few fountain pens. I went to the mall, and when I approached that store, I noticed it was a fancy jewelry and ornament store rather than a pen shop.

When I asked the shopkeeper if they had any fountain pens, he directed me to a showcase in the store, where I found a small collection of pens meant to be carried as decorative items rather than used mainly for writing.

The cost of one of these pens was probably more than the amount needed to buy basic pens or pencils for an entire school. This was when I realized that fountain pens were no longer considered items of essential use but had become antique pieces of vanity.

I looked around the room and also discovered that some other items had a similar fate, such as wristwatches, which were now being used only for presentation while everybody depended on their phones to tell the time.

Fortunately, fountain pens are still being used in some other parts of the world. I purchased a few pens online that came with ink reservoirs called "converters," which were used to draw ink from a traditional ink bottle. I really enjoyed writing with a fountain pen again.

There were days when the ink would smudge on my fingers, but I liked that because it resembled my school years. I got several comments from people admiring my pens, but I realized that in their minds, I was using the pens for extravagance.

However, I was quick to correct them and say that these pens cost me less than the cost of their lunch.

When somebody asked to borrow my pen a few times, I reluctantly gave it to them, worried that they would ruin the nib with their handwriting slant.

Still, it was almost humorous to find out that most millennials don't even know how to hold a fountain pen and could not write properly without scratching the paper.

This is when I started carrying a pen case with the capacity of two pens. I kept my fountain pen in one of the slots and carried a ballpoint pen in the other just in case anybody asked me to lend them a pen to write with.

Medicine is not the only profession that has moved away from handwriting. If you look around, you will see omnipresent examples. You do not have to write many checks anymore because most banking and monetary transfers now occur electronically.

Students have to handwrite less and less each day since most of their work is expected to be submitted online. Students even take notes on their tablets and laptops during class. Bookkeeping for many businesses is now done on electronic spreadsheets.

Appointments for almost anything are made with online software, such as at your hair salon, dentist, or car dealer. Your check at restaurants comes as a printed receipt rather than a handwritten one. A lot of times, you also tip electronically.

You do your taxes online now instead of filling out paper forms and even vote electronically. It is said that a Judge, when delivering a death sentence, would break the pen's nib, signifying the decision's finality.

However, in today's world, where the death penalty is still given, perhaps this is also documented on a computer screen. The list of such examples is long, and it goes on.

It is also interesting how our reflexes have changed. In the handwriting days, the day would start by writing the date at the beginning of each piece of documentation. If somebody asked you what date it was, it would be at the tip of your tongue since you wrote it down numerous times that day.

Now the computer auto-populates the date, and if you are asked what date it is, you have to look at the computer screen or the phone screen to answer.

Similarly, when somebody asked what time it was, the reflex was to look at the clock on the wall or glance at your wristwatch. Now, your hand instantly goes towards your phone screen to see what time it is.

One of the most acclaimed novels of the twentieth century was "*1984*" by George Orwell. In this novel, written in 1949, the writer depicts a fictional dystopian world, many aspects of which still resonate with the current times.

Many words used in the novel have become part of English literature, such as "Big Brother," "Thought police," and "Two Minutes Hate."

However, there are a couple of references to handwriting that are not widely recognized, which I will share with you here.

The protagonist, Winston Smith, uses a device at work into which he speaks, and it automatically transcribes his words onto paper. He calls the device "Speak-write." He calls a pen an "archaic instrument, seldom used even for signatures."

In 1949, this was pure imagination, but in today's world, daily, I dictate all my notes by speaking to a similar device that is connected to the electronic health record.

Closed captioning or subtitles are now available for any TV program, which is also now achieved by automatic speech transcription by software displayed as text at the bottom of the screen.

Now that doctors are not writing as much anymore, these jokes are also fading. I used to be annoyed by a patient, or a friend if they made an illegible handwriting joke with me since I always considered my handwriting not to be as bad.

I enjoyed this expression used by Orwell as a rebuttal to those jokes, which implies that if your brain is functioning at a higher level, you don't give as much attention to the clarity of the handwriting, but if the upper echelons of human intellect are lacking, all the remaining efforts of the brain are consumed at making the handwriting neat and legible!

Ultimately, I request that this not be taken as criticism of modern technology. One should always be open to innovation and embrace it readily while trying to revive tradition until innovation becomes the new tradition.

For those skeptical that handwriting will ever become extinct, please realize the irony that I just wrote a handwriting elegy without handwriting it, and you just finished reading a number of paragraphs typed with a keyboard on a computer screen.

www.ingramcontent.com/pod-product-compliance
Lightning Source LLC
Chambersburg PA
CBHW020406110726
47899CB00006B/1877
9798993882406